Margaret Roberts

Anti-ageing
TISSUE SALTS

Published by Struik Nature
(an imprint of Penguin Random House South Africa (Pty) Ltd)
Reg. No. 1953/000441/07
The Estuaries No. 4, Oxbow Crescent, Century Avenue, Century City, 7441
PO Box 1144, Cape Town, 8000 South Africa

Visit **www.penguinrandomhouse.co.za** and join the Struik Nature Club for
updates, news, events and special offers.

First published in 2016

10 9 8 7 6 5 4 3 2 1

Publisher: Pippa Parker
Managing editor: Helen de Villiers
Editors: Colette Alves, Julia Casciola
Typesetter: Deirdré Geldenhuys
Proofreader: Glynne Newlands

Reproduction by Hirt & Carter Cape (Pty) Ltd

Printed and bound by DJE Flexible Print Solutions, Cape Town, South Africa

Print: 978 1 77584 358 0
ePub: 978 1 77584 359 7
ePDF: 978 1 77584 360 3

Warning: The content of this book is not intended as a substitute for
consultation with a medical professional. Do not undertake any course or
treatment without the advice of your doctor. The author and publishers take
no responsibility for any illness or discomfort that may result from information
contained in this book.

Contents

Preface

My journey with tissue salts began over 50 years ago. As the years pass, I have been surprised over and over again at the versatility of these precious salts, and by the sheer number of ailments and behaviours that can be rectified when one includes them in one's daily health-building routine.

Today the world stands teetering on unreliable supports – stress, anger, despair, illness, deprivation and change engulf every one of us, and we know not which way to turn. Mentally, physically and spiritually we feel bereft of all that was once positive, attainable and rewarding. And so my interest and work began, using the tissue salts to remedy this dis-ease, and to relieve everyday symptoms, as well as the more serious conditions that can come with age.

Organic foods and herbs play a huge role in building health, relieving stress and steadying the body under the pressure of work and increasing years. Within those parameters a fascinating path of discovery unfolded for me. I found new uses for the tissue salts and remarkable new combinations, and together with herbal extracts, they became part of an extraordinary equation that led to this unusual book. I feel that it is one of my most important books, on a subject that we all need to become familiar with. We are ageing too fast, with too much stress and lack of precious time for anything worthwhile, least of all for ourselves.

Included in these pages are the 'super foods' (see p.12), which are rich in the tissue salts (minerals) and vitamins our body requires for optimum health. They slow the ageing process and nourish our bodies, our brains and our outlook. Threaded throughout are also the physical problems we encounter as the years add up, and how the tissue salts can correct, revitalise and steady us, opening new horizons of health and conferring new positivity.

Step by step, the book will guide you along easy paths, introducing the tissue salts and different ways of eating, thinking, cooking and even growing food. Thus you will be familiarised with the vital organic ingredients we need to build health and strength in our senior years. Most of all I want to give you formulas for coping with the stresses and shocks, exhaustion and fears, worries and dilemmas that beset us daily. Tissue salts and living foods and herbs are an inexpensive and easy way to help us cope in this fast-paced changing world of which we are so fragile a part.

I have included a comprehensive alment chart at the end of the book that will allow you to find what you are looking for quickly and easily, and have used my decades of experiences to create combinations that ease our stresses and bring the peace we desire.

I say again, as I did in my first book on tissue salts, that this may be one of the most valuable and unusual books you will ever read, and one of the most significant that I will ever write. I hope that each page will be of benefit to you, and that you will be blessed through the 'golden years' ahead!

MARGARET ROBERTS
The Herbal Centre
De Wildt, North West
South Africa

Introduction

Modern life presents many challenges, decisions, environmental uncertainties and health issues. It is as though challenge is the order of the day, and from midlife onwards this seems to intensify. We need to be steadfast and clear, as the decisions we make daily can affect our future, which appears increasingly uncertain. But with balanced thinking, simple healthy eating, and with the comfort and support of the tissue salts in our daily routine, life becomes stable and joyful!

My long life has been dedicated to working with herbs, healing foods and the wonderful biochemic tissue salts, and this book brings these themes together. My hope is that it will guide readers through a healthy and positive midlife and onward through the senior years, enabling all elderly people to love life and reap the benefit of slowing the ageing process.

I have come to rely on tissue salts and wise eating – and there is no doubt that these two actions build health. Thus, I am ever grateful for the life-changing discovery of Dr Schuessler (1821–1898), an eminent 19th century German physician who discovered that when the human cell was reduced to ashes, 12 minerals remained. He called his method of treatment 'Biochemistry' from the Greek word bios, meaning 'course of life', and 'chemistry', meaning knowledge of the 'elements of life'. Dr Schuessler regarded the inorganic tissue salts as the 'core of wellbeing', and I have found this to be the case.

Included at the back of the book is an ailment index, with the tissue salt number indicating the salt we need to take. Where there are plus signs, this indicates that those specific salts work well together.

When you have a particular condition, it is good practice to re-read all about that specific tissue salt. For example, if you have cramps at night, then re-read the Mag. Phos. chapter, check the foods you need and include those in your diet, and avoid all the danger foods (see p.12). If the symptoms persist, see your doctor. **Self-diagnosis is not recommended, and an annual medical check-up is advised as we age.** Be sure to check your skin for odd spots and dark moles with uneven edges and see a dermatologist if necessary. Have a dental check-up every six months and do not neglect eye and ear health.

I keep all 12 tissue salts on my bathroom shelf, lined up in number order so that they are easy to see and select. I also keep the 'Combin 12' formula, which is all 12 salts in one tablet, for when I am in a hurry and in doubt as to what I need, as well as the combined remedies like 'Flu Remedy', 'Radiation Remedy', 'Arthritis and Gout Remedy', 'Sleepless Remedy', and the precious 'Crisis Remedy'. These are true jewels that immediately calm and ease the situation. Look on tissue salts as 'little lifesavers' and use them with the knowledge that they are safe and effective, and that we all need them in some way or another.

As stress does so much damage, I have worked with special care on the 'stress releasers', and my combination of these vital salts has become a gentle panacea. I have seen it in action in so many instances, from calming a skittish racehorse to soothing an apprehensive child, a lost dog or an agitated 80-year-old moving out of her home. All are calmed and eased, and I thank Dr Schuessler, doctors Carey and Perry who continued his work, and the many brave doctors who have taken the tissue salts forward since then. Today, in the hectic years of the 21st century, the subtle yet profound action of these mineral salts is more needed than they could have known.

As the years accelerate, I look on the tissue salts as something that grounds us as well as easing our tensions and illnesses. I urge everyone to become familiar with them and the foods in which they appear, and hope that this book will be a comforting companion as you negotiate life's challenges and changes.

How tissue salts can help

Deficiency in a specific tissue salt has far-reaching effects. Confusion, reactivity and mood swings all indicate that a specific tissue salt is deficient, and as a consequence life's problems can seem insurmountable. Technology seems to have ushered in a world hovering daily between rage, rudeness and aggression on the one hand and confusion, indecision and anxiety on the other.

I am comforted that by taking Nat. Mur. I can think clearly, and that my mood is lifted. I am grateful to have Kali. Phos. and Calc. Fluor. to give to my grandchildren facing tests, school plays, bullying at school, and the stress of sport's matches. Rushing, anxiety and a fluttering heart seem to be the order of the day and Nat. Mur. and Kali. Phos. calm us all, even the anxious dog, in the midst of a crisis!

A craving for sweets, ice-cream and chocolates can make easy-going children moody and difficult. Nat. Phos. will soothe the tensions quickly, and together with Kali. Phos. a small crisis can be averted! The tissue salts work for everyone, in every age group. They become the friend we need who holds out a steadying hand and gives us that moment of strength to keep on going. They literally help us to feel better and to *be* better!

Why should we take tissue salts?

- Tissue salts quickly replace the lost minerals that our bodies need.
- Our soils are depleted of health-boosting minerals. Chemical fertilisers are being used to sustain commercial food crops, thus we no longer get the necessary minerals through our food. This is the main reason why we need tissue salts.
- Tissue salts reduce stress, panic, fear and over-excitement and release the tension that these feelings generate.
- We no longer eat healthily. Convenience foods, fast foods and processed foods generate cravings in us, and we indulge those cravings. The result is poor health and an increasing need for organically grown food and tissue salts.
- When vital minerals are not replaced, it weakens our resistance to illnesses and afflictions. Fortunately, these conditions can be relieved by using tissue salts.
- Tissue salts build our depleted immune systems and build the brain too. They increase our resistance to infection and help to replenish lost minerals and balance the system.
- They are the most incredible anti-agers. No one can afford to neglect this as we age day by day, accelerating speedily as we pass 50 years – and at breakneck speed after 75!
- Fatigue and exhaustion are so common in our daily lives; however, we can be restored and revitalised directly by the tissue salts. They have an almost immediate calming effect.
- Tissue salts have a profound effect, entirely naturally and with no side-effects. They are rapidly absorbed, non-toxic, non-addictive and can be taken with prescription medication.

Signs of ageing

Old age is not a disease; however, the pace of modern life can cause fatigue, stress and bewilderment in the elderly. Even those in middle age can be overwhelmed, with a subsequent fear of the unknown. Many factors in our daily life accelerate ageing and each one of us needs to consider these and rectify them where possible.

Our new tissue salts

At the beginning of 2016 we completely reformulated our tissue salts into meticulously processed lactose-free tablets and powders, with careful dosages indicated on each bottle.

They are professionally made for us, and we post these beautifully packaged tissue salt tablets, combinations and powders countrywide (contact us on margaretroberts@lantic.net). The combinations are my own tried-and-tested formulas that I have found to be remarkable over the now 50-plus years that I have worked with these precious salts, and I am both comforted and elated that such a superior product can now be offered to everyone under the Margaret Roberts label.

Our tissue salts are contained in dark glass bottles to protect them from light. They are in a non-lactose base and need to dissolve slowly in the mouth to be absorbed. Tip the tablets into the bottle lid so that they are not handled too much. The usual dosage is two tablets sucked slowly every 10 minutes, or hourly as needed.

The tablets can be crushed to add to drinks, teas and healing creams and lotions. Alternatively, we now supply the tissue salts in a finely powdered form, in convenient bottles. A general dose for the powder is half a teaspoon. Remember that this is pure tissue salt, untouched by human hands, and the powder can be dissolved in a little hot water.

Signs of ageing that we will notice include reduced elasticity of the skin and dry skin; changing hormone levels; loss of agility and strength in the legs, making sitting on the ground uncomfortable; increased body fat around the mid-section; decreased bone density; and aching joints and loss of flexibility, which often sets in gradually.

There can also be reduced immunity, and cardiovascular changes such as accelerated heartbeat or circulatory problems. Blood sugar levels need to be checked regularly as we age because there can be changes that we are unaware of. Blood pressure and cholesterol levels can also shift, so get these checked too.

What actually causes ageing?

If we really look at ageing and pinpoint the most common causes, we would come up with processes that we seemingly have little control over, from biological and genetic to environmental. However, by using the tissue salts and regulating our daily diet and lifestyle habits, a lot of the deterioration can be controlled and alleviated. It is certainly worth looking into and worth recording our findings for future reference.

I remember being startled to discover that stress causes the anti-inflammatory and antioxidant defence network to become compromised, accelerating ageing and disease. A chronic, often mild, inflammatory process is therefore an anti-stress response at cellular and molecular level.

Eating processed foods is another trigger, as these foods often contain carcinogenic flavour-enhancers, preservatives, stabilisers and additives that contribute to the inflammatory process. Lack of vitamins and minerals in the diet, large amounts of sugar and salt, skipping meals (which affects blood glucose levels), overeating (which puts stress on the body and increases the number of free radicals), and poor lifestyle habits such as not exercising, late nights and little contact with nature, are all factors in the ageing process. You will realise how much healthier your grandparents were without the 'help' of the food industry, and how they lived with far less stress, often to a ripe old age.

The daily diet

No amount of tissue salts can fully repair the damage done by poor eating and drinking habits. From middle age onwards, every mouthful that goes into our bodies needs to be health building. Become familiar with the health-boosting 'super foods' and the toxic 'danger foods' and plan accordingly.

Meals in our senior years need to be laden with the good vitamins, minerals and nutrients that boost our immune systems and our brains; here is where home-made salads, soups and stews and freshly squeezed juices are our daily health support. If our outlook is positive and we are eating mineral-rich fruits and vegetables, our ageing process will be slow, gentle and rewarding.

Start every morning with a good breakfast, for example, non-instant oats or muesli with banana and goji berries, chopped almonds and a sprinkling of sunflower seeds. Enjoy this with plain unsweetened Bulgarian or Greek yoghurt. Eat a wide variety of foods; as far as possible these should be organically grown, and wherever you can, grow your own. Choose local seasonal produce and in the cold months make warming soups, stews and stir-fries.

Where you need salt, use pink Himalayan salt or plain non-iodised sea salt. To avoid water retention, be aware of the amount of salt you use. Rather use lemon juice, fresh or dried thyme, coriander seeds, and finely chopped celery and celery seeds as a salt substitute and delicious healthy flavouring. Mix these ingredients together and keep them in a jar near the stove for quick sprinkling.

Avoid sugar and sweeteners and replace with fresh or dried stevia leaves (not the processed white powder). This plant is 300 times sweeter than sugar and is safe for diabetics as it does not contain sugar. Rather, it contains 'stevicide', a powerful natural sweetener. Check your tolerance to lactose in dairy products and to gluten in wheat, as this can often change over the years. I have often said that if we exclude sugar, gluten and lactose from our diets for three months, we would see an incredible change in our health.

Drink at least six glasses of filtered water daily, as well as more herbal teas and green teas, and cut down on alcohol and coffee drastically. Avoid any food containing hydrogenated fats. Use extra-virgin cold-pressed olive oil, as it has been used safely and with health benefits for thousands of years. This oil is safe for cholesterol levels too.

We need to eat at least five portions of fresh fruit and vegetables daily. Your salad is a cornerstone here, with abundant greens such as lettuce, parsley and celery being key ingredients. Add grated carrots, beetroot and apple, or cubes of pineapple, chopped green peppers, sweet paprikas and chillies if liked, and whatever is in season. Include sprouts and micro-greens, which are full of enzymes and nutrients, sprinkle fresh herbs over your salad, and make it a daily feast for the whole family!

Be inventive and include the salad ingredients rich in the tissue salt of your choice (there is a list at the end of each chapter). Try growing celery, baby spinach, rocket, peppers and butter lettuce; you will be surprised at how easily they grow. And do not forget the windowsill garden of sprouts and micro-greens. We post seeds for sprouting countrywide and include easy instructions (email: margaretroberts@lantic.net). This can become a fascinating hobby and a profitable one as well, and takes very little effort.

Try to reduce red meat unless you have a source of organically raised mutton or young beef. Find a source of organic chicken, and eat fish three times a week. Plain hake can be made into delicious fish cakes with parsley and celery, or stir-fried with onions and green peppers, and served with home-made oven-baked chips or the much-loved mashed sweet potatoes.

And finally, really get into juicing (vegetables, fruit and greens) – it is the Rolls Royce of healthy eating and will really boost your vitality. Grow wheatgrass and barley grass for this purpose. If possible, read through *My 100 Favourite Herbs*, *Edible and Healing Flowers*, *100 New Herbs*, *Healing Foods* and *Tea*, and become aware of the benefits of living foods rich in tissue salts.

11

Danger foods

- Sugar in all forms, including sweets, chocolates, cakes and ice-cream.
- Sweeteners, other than fresh or dried stevia leaves or a touch of honey.
- Everything 'white': white sugar, icing sugar, white rice, white bread, white flour.
- Everything 'instant': pies, fries, instant soups, instant desserts, instant coffee, instant custard, and bought mayonnaise, sauces, relishes and spreads.
- Processed foods such as prepared meals, which often contain large amounts of salt, sugar and unhealthy fats.
- Processed meats: sausages, salami, Viennas, polony and meat spreads.
- Unhealthy fats, such as heated fats, fried foods and hydrogenated fats.
- Fizzy/carbonated drinks, bottled sweetened juices, and concentrated and pasteurised 'fruit juices'.
- Alcohol.
- Salted snacks: crisps, highly salted nuts, and processed biltong with flavourants and too much salt.
- Preservatives such as benzoic acid, sulphur dioxide and sodium benzoate, which can cause respiratory distress.
- Genetically modified (GM) foods such as canola, maize and soya.

Super foods

- All dark green leafy foods.
- Brightly coloured fresh fruit and vegetables.
- Sprouts and micro-greens.
- Home-made juices full of vitamins, minerals and enzymes, including ingredients such as wheatgrass, cucumber, celery, parsley, carrots, apples and lemons.
- Healthy fats, such as avocados, olives, raw nuts and seeds and cold-pressed olive oil.
- Natural sweeteners such as dates, honey and stevia (fresh or dried, not the processed powder form).

1 Calc. Fluor.

Calcium Fluoride • *Calcarea Fluorata*

Keywords for Calc. Fluor. are 'elasticity' and 'flexibility', as it tones many parts of the body. It is found in the surface of bones, in tooth enamel, in the muscular fibres of the skin, in the blood vessels, as well as in the joints. In other words, the connective tissue of the entire body depends on Calc. Fluor., hence it is vitally important. This exceptional tissue salt is present naturally in organically grown produce, grown in mineral-rich soil.

As we age we seem to become overloaded with information, tensions, pressures and anxieties – even in our 40s. This is where Calc. Fluor. is a beacon of hope. By including it in the daily diet we become more efficient, energetic and positive. I often call it the 'coping salt', because if taken regularly it helps us to 'lighten up' that feeling of not managing. I have noticed that this feeling is more common if one lives in an area that has long days of rain, cold and dark.

The skeleton

Calc. Fluor. strengthens bones and accelerates the healing of fractures; it also strengthens joints, eases discomfort of the lower back, and relieves the deep weariness we so often feel. Remember that the strength of the back is an indicator of how well we manage our daily tasks, our jobs, and even how easily we get in and out of a car.

Take two Calc. Fluor. tablets frequently (also in the case of gouty enlargement of the joints) and alternate with two Nat. Mur. tablets as well as two Silica tablets. This little trio puts the spring back in one's step. As people age, so many lose the joy of the small things we take for granted when younger, such as being pain-free when going up and down steps. Calc. Fluor. preserves the simple pleasure of easy movement. It is also helpful for osteoporosis.

Bones, joints and tendons

In the case of bone 'spurs', especially under the heel, take the homeopathic remedy 'Hekla Lava', and suck two Calc. Fluor. tablets 10 times over the course of the day. Calc. Fluor. is essential for tendons with no elasticity, for tumours on the tendon, and for a 'locked' or hardened tendon. Again, suck two tablets up to 10 times daily to relieve these conditions.

This tissue salt helps to ease carpal tunnel syndrome and bony outgrowths, cysts or injuries on the wrist, as well as pain when writing or using the hands. Calc. Fluor. is also recommended if one elbow is bigger than the other and there is stiffness in the joint, or where there is pain and strain on an elbow.

For a knee that suddenly 'gives way' and does not bear weight, or a joint that slips out of the socket easily, Calc. Fluor. will help, especially if taken 4–6 times through the day. It is also the answer for ligaments and tendons that slip easily and that cannot hold under chiropractic treatment. Slipped discs and pain in the back and neck need Calc. Fluor., and sportsmen and -women will find it a panacea for bone pains.

As a dedicated gardener, I find Calc. Fluor. to be my gardening remedy, especially after digging. When lower back pain engulfs the slightest movement, I make a strong Calc. Fluor. cream to massage into the back; it can also be used on sprained or twisted ankles, sore hips and aching knees. Apply this cream alternately with my much-loved Herbal Heat cream, which can be ordered from the Margaret Roberts Herbal Centre (email: margaretroberts@lantic.net) and will be despatched by post.

Oat straw tea for osteoporosis

Tea made with ripe oat straw is rich in bone-building minerals, including Calc. Fluor., and a cup daily serves as a bone tonic. If possible, grow your own oats. Allow the grain to ripen to a golden colour, then reap and cut into small pieces. Store the straw in airtight tins or jars. To make the tea, pour a cup of boiling water over half a cup of chopped oat straw with a few oat seeds and stir frequently. Strain the tea after five minutes and add four crushed Calc. Fluor. tablets, four Nat. Mur. tablets and a squeeze of lemon juice if liked, and sip slowly.

A similar brew can be used as a cool-drink base. Place two cups of oat straw and two litres of water in a heavy-bottomed pot and simmer for 20 minutes with the lid on. Allow to cool, then strain, pour into a jug and store in the fridge. Use as a cool-drink base by adding unsweetened apple or grape juice and enjoy the bone-building benefits!

Calc. Fluor. massage cream

10 Calc. Fluor. tablets
1 tablespoon hot water
1 cup good aqueous cream
10 drops pure lavender essential oil
10 drops of mint (*Mentha*) essential oil
10 drops rosemary essential oil

Crush the Calc. Fluor. tablets and dissolve in the hot water. Mix into the aqueous cream, then add the lavender, mint and rosemary essential oils, and mix thoroughly. Spoon the cream into a glass jar with a good screw-top lid, and label. Warm the jar in a bowl of hot water before applying the cream. I find that it works especially well after a hot bath.

The eyes

When Calc. Fluor. levels are low in the body, cataracts can form or cyst-like layers of cells on the eye surface known as corneal ulceration. Daily Calc. Fluor. will help, but these conditions need to be checked by an eye specialist.

Flickering flashes of light and blurred vision, a delay when focusing, nervous tics and eye ache all indicate a lack of Calc. Fluor. Take two tablets at least four times a day.

In their early stages, conjunctivitis and cataracts can be 'dissolved' with Calc. Fluor. to a large extent, and an 'eyewash' wiped over the closed eyes is soothing. Dissolve six tablets in half a cup of warm water. Saturate cotton wool pads in the water, squeeze out gently and apply to the eyes. Lie back and relax for 10 minutes and repeat a couple of times. It is wonderfully soothing.

When there is itchiness, irritation and tears, dissolve 10 Calc. Phos. tablets and 10 Nat. Mur. tablets as a wash or eyebath, and take two tablets of each every hour until the condition improves.

Oral health

Calc. Fluor. is much needed if there is dental decay, and when the teeth feel loose in the sockets. In these cases there may also be a dry mouth and translucent tips to the teeth, as well as cracked lips and sores at the corners of the mouth. See your dentist to have these conditions checked.

1 Calc. Fluor.

To make a Calc. Fluor. mouthwash, dissolve six tablets in one cup of hot water and swish it around the mouth, retaining it for as long as is comfortable before swallowing. Do this at least three or four times through the day, and suck two Calc. Fluor. tablets every now and then. This will help to soothe the sensitivity of the teeth and sweeten the breath.

Calc. Fluor. lip cream

Try this cream for dry, cracked lips and corners of the mouth; it is more healing than lip balm.

1 cup good aqueous cream
1 cup pennywort *(Centella asiatica)* leaves
10 Calc. Fluor. tablets, crushed
1 tablespoon hot water
2 teaspoons vitamin E oil

Simmer the aqueous cream and pennywort leaves in a double boiler. Pennywort is an easy-to-grow herb that helps to clear gum infections and bleeding mouth ulcers. Stir the mixture frequently for 20 minutes, then strain and add the crushed Calc. Fluor. tablets dissolved in the tablespoon of hot water. Add the vitamin E oil, mix well, and spoon the cream into a sterilised jar with a good screw-top lid and label. Massage it frequently into the lips.

The respiratory system

I used to be a bad asthmatic until tissue salts changed my breathing patterns in my 30s. I began with Calc. Fluor., which is perfect for an irritating tight cough that leaves one breathless, as well as for postnasal drip and middle-ear infection. Suck two Calc. Fluor. tablets with two Silica tablets 3–6 times a day and be diligent about it.

Coughs, colds and flu that leave a breathless discomfort respond well to Calc. Fluor., usually combined with Silica. 'Grandmother's cough', a tight, breathless cough that most elderly people suffer from, is often triggered by food particles, sharp inhalation of the breath, dust or even a sudden cold draught. Two Calc. Fluor. tablets should be sucked for quick relief.

Calc. Fluor. cream for throbbing haemorrhoids

1 cup good aqueous cream
1 cup fresh pennywort leaves (*Centella asiatica*)
10 tablets each of Calc. Fluor., Kali. Sulph. and Ferrum Phos.

Simmer the aqueous cream and fresh pennywort leaves in a double boiler. Press the leaves and stems down well to release the precious oils. Simmer the mixture for 20 minutes, then cool and strain. Add the crushed Calc. Fluor., Kali. Sulph. and Ferrum Phos. tablets, dissolved in a little hot water. Stir well and spoon into labelled glass jars. Apply frequently, smoothing the cream gently into the affected area. At the same time suck two tablets of each of the three tissue salts three or four times throughout the day. The cream can also be applied as a poultice on a pad of cotton wool to soothe the itching and irritation.

The circulatory system

Varicose veins and painful piles top the list here. Once again, Calc. Fluor. makes an excellent cream, which I make with pennywort in it for physiotherapists when patients are distressed and in discomfort. Calc. Fluor. shrinks and eases protruding piles and tones the area gently.

The digestive system

Suck two Calc. Fluor. tissue salts frequently when there is belching, burping, burning discomfort, hiccups and vomiting up of undigested food. Check the diet when this occurs and make notes to identify patterns. If you experience discomfort after heavy meals, take two or three Calc. Fluor. tablets three times daily.

Today hiatus hernia is a fairly common ailment and distended bowel pockets have also become more prevalent and can lead to irritable bowel syndrome. Two Calc. Fluor. tablets sucked 3–6 times a day is both healing and comforting in the advancing years, and relieves constipation too. Remember that Calc. Fluor. puts elasticity back into the tissues, and in the digestive system this is hugely important.

A soothing digestive tea can be made by pouring a cup of boiling water over two thumb-length sprigs of fresh mint or lemon balm (*Melissa officinalis*). Stir well and strain after five minutes. Add four crushed Calc. Fluor. tablets, stir well to dissolve, and sip slowly. This tea is an excellent bedtime drink to ease the digestive system, and growing both mint and lemon balm is easy (see *My 100 Favourite Herbs*).

Growths, swellings and glands

Be on the lookout for cysts, bumps on or under the skin, over-production of tissue, knotty lymphatic glands, nodules or swollen lymph glands. Two Calc. Fluor. tablets sucked 6–10 times through the day will greatly soothe, shrink and tone the area, similar to how this tissue salt soothes enlarged varicose veins.

Calc. Fluor. also helps with fibroids, cysts in the breasts, Hodgkin's disease and even calcification of the glands. Let your doctor monitor any growths and swellings, and take lots of Calc. Fluor. every day. Where there is a tendency to develop calcium deposits in the ears and the balance is disturbed, try Calc. Fluor. frequently.

The skin

Remember that Calc. Fluor. softens, strengthens and tones, which makes it a really good remedy for cracked heels, rough calluses on hands and feet and for bumps on ageing skin. It is also helpful where there is a tendency to bruise. In addition to the tablets, use the Calc. Fluor. cream (see p.15) on these skin conditions.

The urinary system

As we age, so the bladder weakens and we may need to find the shortest path to the toilet wherever we go! Two Calc. Fluor. tablets sucked at least four times a day will gradually strengthen the bladder and urethra, and in men with an enlarged prostate gland and where there is hardening of the tissues, two or three tablets should be sucked slowly 4–6 times a day, even up to 10 times a day. This helps to soothe the panic, discomfort and irritation. I keep all 12 bottles of tissue salts on a tray on my dressing table for quick access, and replace the bottles regularly as some are used up faster than others, and Calc. Fluor. is one of those quickly used salts.

Often the back is included in bladder weakness; fortunately Calc. Fluor. works on the vertebrae and discs too. On days when there is lots of discomfort and pain, two Calc. Fluor. tablets sucked every hour or so seems to steady and calm, often with Kali. Phos. to lift the spirits. So be sure to have a sufficient supply.

Sleep

Sleep can become elusive as we age, especially when worries and grief beset us. Here is where Silica and Kali. Phos. combined with Calc. Fluor. is such a potent remedy. Anxiety and disturbing dreams can be cleared by taking two Calc. Fluor. and two Kali. Phos. tablets at least five times through the day; before going to bed, take three of each plus two Silica tablets.

Calc. Fluor. and chamomile bedtime tea is calming and instantly soothing should you wake in the night and find getting back to sleep impossible. I grow chamomile every winter and save the flowers, stored in a glass jar, for this safe bedtime brew, but chamomile sachets are available at supermarkets now. Have them available for night-time sleeplessness.

Pour a cup of boiling water over two teaspoons of chamomile flowers or one sachet of chamomile tea. Let the tea draw for five minutes and stir well. Strain and add four crushed Calc. Fluor. tablets, four crushed Kali. Phos. tablets and two crushed Silica tablets. Stir well, sip slowly and sleep tight!

How you feel

As we age worries can engulf us and life seems to change too fast, with problems constantly calling for attention. For others, life can seem like a silent void. Either way we are affected to some degree. Depression, irritation, short temper, helplessness, hopelessness, lack of concentration, sadness, instability, erratic behaviour, quickness to blame others and a restless, demotivated disposition can overwhelm us.

We need to remember how important Calc. Fluor. is and take it several times a day. It helps us to concentrate, to stabilise, to cope and to remain calm. Often those who need Calc. Fluor. have a fear of poverty and work tremendously hard, investing carefully and worrying a lot. People who are very anxious, organised and systematic typically need Calc. Fluor.

To make a good drinking water for all the above conditions, dissolve two Calc. Fluor. tablets, two Kali. Phos. tablets and two Silica tablets in each glass of filtered drinking water. The mood will brighten, worries will lift, a happier person will appear, bone and tooth problems will disappear, and cysts and hardened tonsils and lymph glands will soften!

Secondary and complementary tissue salts

Silica works very well with Calc. Fluor. This combination is particularly effective for fortifying the bones. Kali. Phos. is also a good secondary or complementary salt to Calc. Fluor., helping with toning, and mental upliftment and brightening. Add two tablets of each when taking Calc. Fluor.

1 Calc. Fluor.

Herbs that contain Calc. Fluor.

The following herbs are easy to grow and should be included in the diet for their Calc. Fluor. content.

Buckwheat (*Fagopyrum esculentum*): The heart shape of the leaves and seeds indicates that buckwheat is a heart and circulation herb. It is rich in many minerals including Calc. Fluor. and is easy to sprout and grow, so include it in the diet often. Ground buckwheat flour can be purchased to make pancakes, biscuits and rusks.

Chickweed (*Stellaria media*): A little winter annual weed, with a high Calc. Fluor. content and the tiniest white flowers, chickweed is much needed for aches and pains, gout and rheumatism, and kidney and bladder problems. Its luscious little leaves are delicious chopped in salads, and it softens the skin and lessens crusty build-up. I use it in creams and lotions and find it wonderfully soothing. Chickweed comes up in the cooler months in most gardens, so look out for it.

Chives (*Allium schoenoprasum*): This herb is one of nature's antibiotics; it also stimulates the immune system. Along with garlic and combined with parsley, it makes a superb salad ingredient that boosts the circulation and assists in building resistance to infections.

Garlic (*Allium sativum*): As we age, garlic becomes more important in our diet. Garlic lowers high blood pressure and high cholesterol. It is a natural antibiotic that kills a broad range of bacteria, as well as protecting the body and boosting the immune system. If you do not like the potent smell, take it in capsule form with parsley.

Mustard plant (*Brassica nigra; Brassica/Sinapis alba*): Green mustard leaves and flowers are a tasty salad ingredient, rich in Calc. Fluor., and the seeds ground with olive oil and honey make a delicious spread or dressing much loved by the elderly. Mustard is a circulatory herb and a member of the brassica family, and it is easy, quick and rewarding to grow as a windowsill crop. It makes a delicious sprout.

Parsley (*Petroselinum crispum*): Long underestimated, parsley is a truly valuable herb, hugely important for the kidneys and for bladder, urinary and prostate problems. It is an excellent detoxifier, so sprinkle home-grown parsley generously on your food, even on scrambled eggs at breakfast time! Have it daily, if possible, and preferably grow your own organic parsley.

Sage (*Salvia officinalis*): Sage is a wonderful herb that clears coughs, flu, colds and bronchitis. It is worth growing for easy teas. Pour a cup of boiling water over ¼ cup fresh leaves and let the tea stand for five minutes, stirring often. Strain and sweeten with a touch of honey if liked and a squeeze of lemon.

Winter savory (*Satureja montana*): A digestive herb, winter savory clears the throat, lungs and sinuses, and eases muscular aches and even constipation. Include it in soups, stews, stir-fries and as a salad dressing chopped into a little lemon juice and olive oil. It is an old-fashioned herb but so rich in Calc. Fluor. that we need to know it and grow it!

Grow your own energy boosters

Buckwheat and mustard are both quick and easy-to-grow salad plants. They are rich in vitamins and minerals, boosting the entire system with their chlorophyll-rich nutrients. The flowers and young succulent seeds are edible and can be made into an energy-boosting salad with lemon juice, chopped parsley, celery and chives. You can also grow these as sprouts.

Foods rich in Calc. Fluor.

Firstly, avoid processed meats, fried foods and too much salt, and avoid all sugar except a touch of honey every now and then. Avoid alcohol, carbonated drinks, energy drinks, colourants, preservatives and chemicals.

Include some of these valuable Calc. Fluor. foods daily: pumpkin, squash, gem squash, marrows, the cabbage family, especially kale, and the onion family (all onions such as spring onions, Welsh onions, garlic, red onions as well as all the other easy-to-grow onions). Grow them in richly composted soil with rock dust, which is literally tissue salts for plants. Also include grapes, oranges, naartjies, lemons and clementines in your diet, and replace wheat flour with rye flour to make bread and rolls, and use rye or buckwheat flour in baking.

Sesame seeds are rich in Calc. Fluor., as well as many other vitamins and minerals. Spinach, broccoli, grapes, vine tips and young vine leaves all contain bioflavonoids and help to elasticise, tone and strengthen cells as the body absorbs their Calc. Fluor. content.

The pith of lemons and oranges is also rich in this tissue salt, and a mere teaspoonful of pith a day, scraped from the inside of the fruit skin, will help nails, skin, teeth and bones to grow beautifully. It also strengthens blood vessel walls and clears the sinuses, and ear, nose and throat blockages.

I find it interesting that if the diet lacks these herbs and foods, all the Calc. Fluor. symptoms appear, unmistakably and clearly! We can correct even a small niggle with the right tissue salt. As we age it is critical to maintain that wellness margin, and we can do so by including at least 60–80% of these foods and herbs in our daily diet, preferably organically grown at home!

Pumpkin fritters

Every year I grow the big, flat white 'boerpampoen' – that staple winter vegetable that keeps well for many months and is loved by South African farmers. This traditional dish must be one of the most enjoyed Calc. Fluor.-rich foods.

1 egg, beaten
1 teaspoon baking powder
Himalayan salt to taste
2 tablespoons flour
2 cups cooked mashed pumpkin (steaming retains the vitamins and minerals)
Olive oil
Ground cinnamon
Honey
Lemon juice

Mix the egg, baking powder, salt and flour into the mashed pumpkin. Heat a little olive oil in a non-stick pan (do not use Teflon-coated pans – we use stainless steel, ceramic-coated pans). Drop spoonfuls of the pumpkin mixture into the pan and fry on both sides until golden brown. Allow the fritters to stand on paper towel to remove any excess oil. Then dust with a little cinnamon and add a touch of honey. Serve hot with a squeeze of lemon juice.

Calc. Fluor. health juice

SERVES 1–2

2 organically grown oranges, peeled
2 apples, peeled
2 carrots, scrubbed
2 cups washed red grapes (if in season)
1 cup fresh parsley
1 cup fresh buckwheat leaves and flowers

Push everything through a juicer, alternating with the buckwheat greens and parsley. Drink immediately. It makes a very refreshing lunch or afternoon drink.

Spinach, broccoli and kale stir-fry

This is a really fantastic and tasty health booster.

1 large onion, finely sliced
2 or 3 tablespoons olive oil
2 cups broccoli florets, broken into small pieces
2 cups finely shredded kale
2 cups shredded spinach
Juice of 1 lemon
1 teaspoon grated lemon rind
1 or 2 tablespoons toasted sesame seeds
Himalayan salt and freshly ground black pepper
Sliced mushrooms (optional)
1 cup grated mozzarella cheese (optional)

In a large pan, stir-fry the onion in a little olive oil until it starts to brown. Then quickly stir-fry the broccoli florets, kale and spinach with the lemon juice and rind. Add the sesame seeds, salt and black pepper and stir-fry briskly, mixing everything together well. Add a touch of water if it looks too dry to soften the vegetables. If you're adding mushrooms, do so now. For extra flavour, add mozzarella cheese as you serve it.

2 Calc. Phos.

Calcium Phosphate • Phosphate of Lime • Calcarea Phosphoricum

This is a real anti-ageing tissue salt, as it builds cells, supports growth, and develops teeth, nails, bones and strength. In addition, it has a wonderful tonic action that nourishes, restores and supports recuperation, particularly in the years beyond midlife. Because of the amazing strength it gives us, we all need to take it daily and include foods rich in Calc. Phos. in our daily diet. The changes are very satisfying!

I often think of Calc. Phos. as a mould or 'matrix', as calcium is the mineral base for growth and development. In the ancient texts this precious mineral is recorded as being particularly valuable for infants, developing children, teenagers and the elderly. It is as important during growth spurts in children as it is for the faltering pain-filled steps of their grandparents, and for all bone pains in between!

What I perhaps appreciate most is that Calc. Phos. helps you get more out of your food, as it is a strong and effective processor, and it also happily gives that 'get-up-and-go' feeling. When you feel a lack of willpower and energy, or a sense of being overwhelmed by life and unable to process it, suck two Calc. Phos. tablets slowly early on in the day and several times through the day. You will notice a pleasant pace picking up with the energy that comes, as well as new positivity and ideas, while the irritability and indecision fall away!

Interestingly, when there is a craving for bacon, salami and salty smoked meats, this is a clear indication that Calc. Phos. is deficient in the body. Other symptoms include white spots on the nails and there may also be a craving for tobacco and cigarettes. In these cases, increase the daily Calc. Phos. intake. Make a cup of chamomile tea, dissolve 10 Calc. Phos. tablets in it, and sip it slowly before going to bed. Start each morning by eating foods that are rich in Calc. Phos., especially a bowl of oats porridge with a few strawberries or figs sliced into it, topped with plain Bulgarian yoghurt and a little honey or fresh chopped stevia leaves for sweetness.

The skeleton

Calc. Phos. is good for strengthening bones and easing stiff joints in older people. It is excellent for those who enjoy sport, especially running and weightlifting, and for ageing athletes.

As Calc. Phos. is essential for strong bones, this tissue salt is particularly important during and after the menopause, when two tablets should be taken 4–6 times a day. It is easily assimilated and helps to build bone and prevent osteoporosis. I am surprised that Calc. Phos. is not prescribed for all over 50 year olds, as it helps us to assimilate calcium-rich foods.

In the case of bone diseases, two Calc. Phos. tablets should be sucked 6–10 times a day. Curvature of the spine can be helped significantly with daily Silica and Calc. Phos. For numbness and for chilliness of aching bones, never forget the power of a hot-water bottle and a hot cup of Calc. Phos. and Ferrum Phos. (six tablets of each dissolved in a cup of hot water and sipped slowly). When there are ulcers and abscesses on the bones or joints, coupled with restlessness, this wonderful formula is a standby, as the salts go to work cleaning and repairing the deep inflammation. As people age, this is needed almost daily. In the case of aching joints, add six Silica tablets too, as this will ease the inflammation and pain.

Slow-healing fractures need Calc. Phos. five or six times a day, and for aches and pains, rheumatism and poor circulation to the bones, suck two tablets at least three times a day to ease things. Remember that this is one of the most useful pain treatments for ageing animals too. Also include MSM (methylsulfonylmethane), a natural painkiller that works well with tissue salts and is available from pharmacies. Take one or two tablets daily with breakfast (it also safe for animals).

The eyes

As we age our eyes can become oversensitive to light. Pink eye (conjunctivitis), eye twitches and flashing lights in the peripheral vision can leave us feeling anxious, but Calc. Phos. comes to the rescue easily.

Calc. Phos. is also known for its role in cataract prevention, for easing aching stiffness behind the eyeball, and for red, irritated eyes. In these cases suck two Calc. Phos. tablets 4–6 times through the day. This will be instantly soothing.

As a young physiotherapist I worked with a knowledgeable Swiss doctor who had grown up with Dr Schuessler's tissue salts. He told me about the compresses his grandmother made for him as a child when he had red, sore, tired eyes. This remedy is also beneficial when one sees flashing lights and when there is eye strain after too much computer work.

Calc. Phos. eye compress

10 Calc. Phos. tablets
½ cup lukewarm water
2 cotton wool pads

Dissolve the tablets in the warm water. Dip the cotton wool pads in the water, wring them out gently, and apply to closed eyes while lying flat. Be sure to have a warm, light blanket on hand, as the aim is to keep comfortable and relaxed. Two tablets can be sucked while resting.

Eye pillow
Try this remedy for aching eyeballs and a cold feeling behind the eyes.

17 x 8cm piece of soft, silky fabric
¾ cup linseeds (flaxseeds)

Sew the fabric into a small rectangular pillow case, leaving a small opening in one corner. Insert a funnel into the opening, pour the linseeds in, and sew the space closed. Lie down flat and place the eye pillow over the eyes. It should feel soft and light. If it feels too heavy, undo a few stiches in the corner and shake out some seeds. The intention of an eye pillow is to feel a gentle pressure over the eyes, which relieves tired eyes after too much computer work or close reading.

Oral health

We need to look after our teeth throughout life, but particularly as we age. Gum disease is more prevalent in the advanced years and can be an indication of heart problems, so visit your dentist at least every six months.

Calc. Phos. is important for strong teeth and a sturdy jaw bone, and two tablets sucked two or three times a day does a valuable job of repairing the mouth and tongue, and remedying pale sensitive gums and tooth decay. A combination of Calc. Fluor. and Calc. Phos. also gives sure, quick results and a dose two or three times a day will clear minor mouth problems and help to heal bleeding gums. Make a Calc. Phos. mouthwash by dissolving 10 Calc. Phos. tablets in a cup of warm water, and swish it around your mouth gently.

I have found my own non-lactose tissue salts easy to use and safe. When tablets made with lactose are left in the mouth (such as when one falls asleep), the lactose can soften tender spots on the teeth, so be sure to dissolve all tissue salts under the tongue and rinse the mouth 30 minutes later.

Calc. Phos. circulation cream

1 cup fresh pennywort *(Centella asiatica)* leaves and stalks
1 cup good aqueous cream
10 Calc. Phos. tablets
1 tablespoon hot water
2 teaspoons vitamin E oil
1 teaspoon lemon essential oil
1 teaspoon tea tree essential oil

Simmer the pennywort and aqueous cream in a double boiler for 30 minutes. Press the leaves firmly and frequently against the sides of the pot to release the oils. Stir thoroughly, then strain through a new sieve and add the Calc. Phos. tablets dissolved in the hot water. Stir well, and add the vitamin E oil, lemon essential oil and tea tree essential oil and mix thoroughly. Spoon the cream into sterilised glass jars with screw-top lids, label and store in a dark cupboard. Apply the cream after a hot bath; warm it beforehand by standing the jar in a bowl of very hot water. Do this each night, especially if you have been standing a lot throughout the day.

The circulatory system

When Calc. Phos. is deficient or even non-existent in the body, chilblains, cold hands and feet, cramps in the legs and feet, and numbness of the feet and hands are likely to occur. These are truly the classic signs of Calc. Phos. deficiency. I make a Calc. Phos. cream for these conditions and find it very helpful when massaged into the feet and lower legs every night after a hot bath. The cream includes pennywort, as it is the best circulatory herb (you can read more about pennywort in *My 100 Favourite Herbs*).

In addition, suck two Calc. Phos. tablets at least 4–6 times a day to relieve the numbness, coldness and poor circulation, and have a cup or two of pennywort tea daily. To make the tea, pour a cup of boiling water over ¼ cup fresh pennywort leaves. Let it stand for five minutes, stir well, strain and sip slowly. A slice of fresh lemon or ginger root is very pleasant in the tea, which can be sweetened with a fresh stevia leaf or a touch of honey. Make it a general rule to have herb teas for 10 days, then take a break for two or three days, and resume for 10 days. This is the most reliable way of getting the most benefit from the herb that the body can process. The power of herbs is exceptional, so use with care.

The digestive system

Calc. Phos. deserves special mention here as it is so helpful with several digestive conditions. Diarrhoea with accompanying colic and bloating, the unsuccessful desire to pass a stool, itching haemorrhoids, anal fissures and cracks, pain in the stomach and colon after eating, and vomiting, colic pains and belching are all eased by Calc. Phos. Suck two tablets every 10 minutes to aid the assimilation of food until symptoms are relieved.

Combine two tablets each of Calc. Phos., Mag. Phos. and Nat. Phos. to ease burning indigestion, belching, gas build-up, flatulence, acidity, spasm, bloating and discomfort throughout the digestive system.

Calc. Phos. will ease irritable bowel syndrome when taken in conjunction with Kali. Phos. and Nat. Sulph., and this precious formula will also help to curb the craving for salty crisps and foods. Learn to make healthier salty snacks such as home-made root crisps. Cut thin slices of sweet potato, butternut and beetroot, spray them lightly with olive oil and season them with Himalayan salt, fresh chopped thyme and coriander seeds. Place the slices on a roasting tray and roast in a medium oven until lightly browned.

Slimming

As people age they seem to need more 'comfort food', which can increase weight and put strain on weight-bearing joints. Calc. Phos. and Calc. Fluor. are the two tissue salts needed to shift excess weight, as they quell the appetite. Two tablets of each, six times daily, will help to calm any obsession with food.

The skin

The skin suffers when there is a lack of Calc. Phos. – it tends to look pale, pasty and generally unhealthy, often with underlying spots and adult acne. Make a lotion to wipe the face and clear the skin, and suck two Calc. Phos. tablets at least four times a day.

Calc. Phos. skin lotion

10 tablets each of Calc. Phos., Nat. Phos. and Ferrum Phos.
1 cup hot water
1 cup pennywort tea, strained (made by infusing a cup of
    pennywort leaves in a cup of boiling water)

Dissolve the tissue salt tablets in the hot water and add the pennywort tea. Use the cooled lotion as a spritz-spray on the face, neck and chest, or wipe it over the skin using cotton wool pads. Discard each pad as you wipe in one direction and use fresh pads frequently. Drink a cup of pennywort tea (see p.28) every day with Calc. Phos., Ferrum Phos. and Nat. Phos. (two tablets of each) dissolved in it. Also suck two tablets of each at least four times a day. This anti-ageing beauty treatment should be applied daily if possible!

How you feel

As people age there can be more complaining, fussiness, frustration and general discontent. Two Calc. Phos. and two Nat. Mur. tablets held in the mouth will start to lift the spirits and the feelings quite magically. To shift moods, I rely on a combination of Kali. Phos., Calc. Phos. and Nat. Mur.; two tablets of each should be sucked frequently. This amazing trio can diffuse many difficult situations, so keep the bottles close at hand. Over the years I have sat through many boardroom meetings wishing that I could slip these three tissue salts into the coffee cups of impossible members!

Calc. Phos. helps with frequent sighing, lack of sleep, and with deep grief, despair and desperation at life generally. When a deep breath is not enough, when the desire to weep is strong and there is an impulse to give voice to your frustrations, reach for Kali. Phos. and Calc. Phos. and suck two tablets of each frequently.

2 Calc. Phos.

Other ailments

When there is a tendency to get coughs, colds, flu and sore throats easily, Calc. Phos. serves as a general immune booster and is very comforting. Suck two tablets twice daily. If you cannot manage to do everything that needs to be done, you feel sluggish and it is easier to say 'no', then Calc. Phos. will become a great friend! It will clear sweaty palms, the desire for a cigarette, and sweating from the head at night; it will also boost the immune system, soothe menopause problems and help with weight loss due to grief or intense stress. Three or four tablets sucked three or four times a day will ease all these difficulties. Place the tablets under the tongue and suck slowly, with long, slow breaths. This is the way to get optimal interaction through the membranes of the mouth.

In the case of a feeling of suffocation due to enlargement of the goitre, six Nat. Mur. and six Calc. Phos. tablets dissolved in hot water and sipped slowly will ease the crisis. This combination also helps with hoarseness, coughing and throat clearing (such as during public speaking), and can be alternated with Calc. Phos. and Ferrum Phos. In my many years of public speaking I have learned to keep a glass of water with 10 tablets each of Calc. Phos., Ferrum Phos. and Nat. Mur. dissolved in it, and to sip it frequently to clear a frog in the throat, burning throat and postnasal drip.

Secondary and complementary salts

Mag. Phos. and Calc. Phos. really enhance each other's effects. If you include Silica, the three become the building or structural salts that give the body strength, vitality and energy. These three tissue salts distribute calcium around the body, refining and building it. Remember that the older we get, the more we need calcium and the foods that contain it.

Kali. Mur. taken with Calc. Phos. is excellent for recovery from bronchitis and pneumonia; when they are combined with Mag. Phos., the brain starts to become clearer, the person calmer and more positive, and moodiness, aggressiveness, fretfulness, peevishness and incoherent thoughts are replaced with co-operation and positivity. This formula can also be used during times of change, grief, memory loss, fear, despair, depression, and helplessness with heart palpitations. It will relieve all of the above and allow positive ways of coping.

The combination of Kali. Mur., Calc. Phos. and Ferrum Phos. improves circulatory weakness and chilliness. Mag. Phos. and Nat. Mur. are also good companions, and they combine well with Ferrum Phos. for vertigo and bleeding gums.

Herbs that contain Calc. Phos.

Grow the herbs below in your garden, as they are so valuable in teas and added to cooked foods and salads. A Calc. Phos. garden is a fabulous way to utilise 'nature's pantry' in its incredible abundance.

Borage (*Borago officinalis*): Rich in calcium, borage can be taken as a tea to treat coughs and the feverish stages of pneumonia, bronchitis and flu. Borage tea mixed with honey and lemon juice is excellent for the throat and chest.

Chamomile *(Matricaria/Chamomilla recutita)*: This herb is rich in Calc. Phos. and makes a delicious tea at the end of a busy day. The tea is calming, unwinding and repairing, and is beautifully suitable as we advance in years. It helps to clear kidney ailments, strengthen the circulation and to ease the digestion. Chamomile is a winter herb, so sow the seed at the end of each summer.

Comfrey (*Symphytum officinale*): Known as 'knit-bone', comfrey helps to knit broken bones, and it clears chest ailments such as pneumonia and bronchitis. Rich in Calc. Phos., the herb helps to relieve backache and kidney infections, and it is a potent anti-ager. To relieve pain, have a cup of comfrey tea once or twice a day for 2–7 days. To mend bones, sip one cup a day, then take a break before continuing as needed, but only briefly. Doctors advise against taking comfrey internally, so consult with your doctor before taking this herb.

Dandelion (*Taraxacum officinale*): I was once advised to eat three dandelion leaves a day to ensure strong bones, teeth, nails and cartilage. I still try to do so and always have plants nearby. Dandelion is a rich source of Calc. Phos., so we need it daily!

Lucerne/Alfalfa (*Medicago sativa*): The succulent green tips of the long stems are delicious in salads, stir-fries, soups and stews, and the flowers are edible too. Lucerne is a real vitality booster, clearing infection and repairing the circulation, and it is an easy-to-grow perennial. It is full of Calc. Phos., as well as vitamins and minerals.

Oats (*Avena sativa*): Use the big-grain non-instant oats to make porridge daily. Oats are high in Calc. Phos. and make a rich restorative tonic and antidepressant; they also build bone and reduce high cholesterol. Use dried ripe oat stems to make teas for osteoporosis and bone building. As we age, this tea becomes increasingly important and valuable (see recipe on p.14).

Breakfast energy booster

SERVES 1–2

This breakfast is packed with energy and will put a spring in your step.

1 cup large flake non-instant oats
1½ cups water
Pinch of Himalayan salt
2 tablespoons sliced strawberries, raspberries, mulberries or cherries
½ cup plain Bulgarian yoghurt
½ cup low-fat milk
1 tablespoon chopped almonds, sunflower seeds and cranberries

Simmer the oats, water and salt gently in a pot, stirring frequently until cooked. Stir in the berries and spoon into a bowl. Add the yoghurt, milk, almonds, sunflower seeds and cranberries. Stir it well and chew it thoroughly. You can also add other nuts and sesame seeds.

Foods rich in Calc. Phos.

We need to include at least eight of these foods in our daily diet. Grow as many as you can and make soups, stews and salads frequently with this nourishing collection.

Green leafy vegetables are a wonderful source of Calc. Phos. Grow a variety of lettuces, spinaches, Chinese greens, cabbages, broccoli and dandelions in your garden for quick picking. Carrots, lentils and cucumbers are also a rich source, and sesame seeds are easy to grow, pretty and packed with calcium.

Strawberries, cranberries, goji berries, mulberries, raspberries, silver cane berries, figs, plums and almonds are all rich in this tissue salt, and make a delicious addition to the diet. Oats and barley are also vital Calc. Phos. sources (remember to make barley water from pearled barley).

Grow your own sprouts, especially lucerne (alfalfa) sprouts, lentil sprouts, oat sprouts, as well as wheat and barley grass for juicing.

Include plain Bulgarian yoghurt in the diet, as well as low-fat cottage cheese, butter, and if possible a little milk (many people are lactose intolerant, so be careful) as they are all good sources of this mineral salt. Grilled lean meat, mutton stews and soft-boiled eggs are high in Calc. Phos. too, so vary the diet and concentrate on these super foods for your health's sake.

Lunchtime health salad

This is a real super salad and will become a favourite quick dish that you can enjoy often.

2 cups young lettuce leaves
1 cup grated carrots
1 cup cooked lentils
1 cup alfalfa sprouts
1 cup wheat sprouts – 3 days old
4 or 5 chopped dandelion leaves
½–1 cup chunky plain cottage cheese
2 sliced hard-boiled eggs
Chopped parsley
Himalayan salt and ground black pepper
Juice of 1 lemon

On a salad platter, lay out the lettuce leaves, then add the grated carrots and lentils mixed with the sprouts, then the chopped dandelion leaves. Add small spoonfuls of the cottage cheese, and the sliced hard-boiled eggs. Sprinkle with chopped parsley, a grinding of Himalayan salt, a touch of black pepper and a squeeze of fresh lemon juice. This salad never tires the palate.

'A salad a day keeps the doctor away' is the new mantra! To give this salad a festive spin over the Christmas holidays, add fresh pineapple slices and figs.

3 Calc. Sulph.

Calcium Sulphate • Sulphate of Lime • Plaster of Paris • Gypsum • *Calcarea Sulphurica*

This is a vital salt in its role as cleanser, purifier and eliminator, and yet it is the least-used of all the tissue salts. It is found in the blood, connective tissue, liver and bile, and also in the epithelial cells in the skin. Taking Calc. Sulph. after Silica to eliminate build-up after coughs, colds and flu, for example, will clear out the mucus thoroughly!

Drs Carey and Perry (who continued Dr Schuessler's work on tissue salts) found Calc. Sulph. to be the great cleanser of chronic infections, which occur when catarrh, inflammatory conditions, slow-healing wounds and bronchial mucus remain around too long. Calc. Sulph. was found to be so remarkable in its action that they called it 'The Biochemical Surgeon'.

Drs Carey and Perry recorded many more facts on the remarkable cleansing action of this salt, particularly with regard to boils, infected acne, ulcers, abscesses and mucus congestion, as well as burning eczemas that are dry and sensitive, and unhealthy skin with infected spots and oily patches. I find it particularly valuable as a 'cleanser' in a healing cream (see p.35) on slow-healing sores such as those that occur in HIV/AIDS, and on infected acne that leaves scars.

Foods rich in Calc. Sulph. should be included in our daily diet because as we age it is harder to clear even simple ailments, which is where Calc. Sulph. is so important. Lotions, washes and creams can all be made easily with Calc. Sulph.-rich herbs and extracts.

Whenever I hear the word 'infection' I reach for Calc. Sulph., as it is multi-beneficial for all infections. This is also why I grow red clover abundantly; it is rich in Calc. Sulph. and makes an exceptional cleansing tea. To make it, pour a cup of boiling water over ¼ cup red clover leaves (and flowers if it is summer). Let the tea stand for five minutes, stir thoroughly, then strain, add six crushed Calc. Sulph. tablets and sip slowly. It will heal difficult infections and clear old coughs and worn-out cells. Make this tea a ritual and it will rebuild your body into enviable 'wellness'! I make it at least twice a week, and include Calc. Sulph. foods in my daily diet.

Calc. Sulph. and Silica healing cream

1 cup stinging nettle tops
1 cup fresh red clover leaves and flowers
1½ cups good aqueous cream
10 tablets each of Calc. Sulph. and Silica, crushed

Simmer the nettle, clover and aqueous cream in a double boiler for 20 minutes, stirring frequently. Set the mixture aside to cool with the lid on. Strain, discard the herbs, and mix in the crushed Calc. Sulph. and Silica tablets. Spoon the mixture into a sterilised jar and label. Use this cream directly on scratches, grazes, infected skin and insect bites. Always wash your hands thoroughly before applying the cream or use a sterilised spatula.

The skin

The first things that draw attention to the skin are pimples, acne, weals, itchy spots and suppurating sores of any size. I learned early on in my original tissue salt studies that Calc. Sulph. was the first remedy to clear any skin 'eruption', even infected mosquito bites. I apply it as a paste, made by dissolving four crushed Calc. Sulph. tablets in a little hot water.

Oats are excellent on oily problem skin, and adult-onset pustular acne can be soothed and healed with an oatmeal paste. Grind a cup of the big, flat, non-instant oat flakes and mix with 10 crushed Calc. Sulph. tablets and enough hot (boiled) water to make a comfortable paste, and apply warm to the area. Work it in gently with the fingers and leave it on for 30 minutes if possible. Wash off with a warm lotion of Calc. Sulph. and red clover.

In a similar way one can also make a gentle oatmeal and Calc. Sulph. scrub to clean acne and improve circulation. Use two cups of dry oats and 20 crushed Calc. Sulph. tablets, well mixed, and store in a screw-top jar. To make the scrub, shake the dry mixture thoroughly, then pour out half a cup and mix into ¾ cup water to make a paste. Use it as a gentle scrub over the acne area as this will improve the circulation.

The eyes

Calc. Sulph. is excellent for conjunctivitis (pink eye) and other eye infections. Crush and dissolve 10 Calc. Sulph. tablets in a cup of hot water, then soak a cotton wool pad in the lotion, squeeze it gently and wipe over closed eyes. It is also wonderfully soothing as a warm

Calc. Sulph. and red clover lotion

1 cup fresh red clover leaves, stems and flowers
1 litre water
10 crushed Calc. Sulph. tablets

Simmer the red clover and water in a heavy-bottomed stainless steel pot for 20 minutes (keep the lid on). Set the mixture aside to cool to a comfortable warmth. Strain and add the Calc. Sulph. tablets and stir thoroughly. Use as a wash or spritz-spray. This is an excellent lotion for rashes, grazes, insect bites and itchy scalp. Grow red clover close to the kitchen so that you can pick it frequently. It is so comforting for these skin conditions, as well as for heat rash and blind pimples under the beard after shaving, that I am even experimenting with red clover soap!

compress. Where there is a yellow discharge in the corners of the eyes, use the pad to wipe it away, discard it and use a fresh one, repeating until the discharge is cleared.

The lotion will also help with minor irritations on the cornea and should be applied as above, morning and evening. For watery eyes and continual tears, suck two Calc. Sulph. tablets 3–6 times during the day to soothe and ease any discomfort. Do this at least twice daily until the symptoms clear.

The ears

In the case of blocked ears, ringing in the ears and continual wax production with earache (check if the wax is dark and see a doctor), suck two Calc. Sulph. tablets up to six times a day. Apply the same lotion as for the eyes, using a pad of cotton wool to wipe the outer ear and to clear the wax gently.

Oral health

When there are bleeding gums, mouth ulcers and gum boils, dissolve 10 Calc. Sulph. tablets in a cup of hot water and use it as a mouth wash; retain the fluid in the mouth for as long as is comfortable before spitting it out. Also suck two or three Calc. Sulph. tablets six times a day and keep them in the mouth for as long as possible, as this will help to clear the infection quickly. Include two Ferrum Phos. tablets with this treatment daily to help fight any new infections.

The circulatory system

I have come to look on Calc. Sulph. as a cleanser and detoxifier for slow-healing and painful varicose veins and for throbbing varicosities, along with cold feet. Two Calc. Sulph. tablets sucked frequently will ease the pain and discomfort and even relieve a throbbing headache. When there are aching lower limbs and burning feet, suck two Calc. Sulph. tablets every 15 minutes or every hour to bring relief. Ulcerated varicosities are painful and fragile, and here is where a cream made with Calc. Sulph. is so helpful.

Slow-healing boils on the legs, in the groin and in the hip joint can be difficult, so be sure to have Calc. Sulph. on hand. Ulcers on the legs often take a long time to heal due to poor circulation. Make the Calc. Sulph. cream (see p.35) and use it to massage the feet and lower legs, and take pennywort tea (see p.28). You will find that cracked heels and dry skin will improve as well, as the circulation improves. Massage the cream into the heels all through winter.

The respiratory system

A persistent sore throat and lingering chesty cough will benefit from Calc. Sulph. and Kali. Sulph. Together, they will clear the infection, ease tonsillitis and clear ongoing discharge from the nose and throat. Suck two tablets of each 4–6 times a day to clear things. As you age, it is vital to keep your doctor aware of how you are feeling, so check in with your practitioner at regular intervals.

To break the pattern of frequent coughs and colds, take two Calc. Sulph. and two Ferrum Phos. tablets three or four times daily during winter. However, where there is serious respiratory infection, follow your doctor's advice and take the tissue salts as a complementary treatment to the medication prescribed.

Olive leaf tea and avocado leaf tea are both a boon for the respiratory system and should be taken twice daily. To make either of these teas, pour a cup of boiling water over ¼ cup fresh torn-up leaf, stir thoroughly and press to release the healing oils and juices from the leaf. Add six crushed Calc. Sulph. tablets to the tea and sip it slowly.

The asthma tree also offers a comforting treatment for tight wheeziness, difficulty breathing and an excess of mucus. Make a tea from the leaves as described above. This plant is fairly bitter, but it can be lessened by removing the midrib from the leaf (see more about this herb in *100 New Herbs*).

3 | Calc. Sulph.

The digestive system

If you suffer from a stomach ulcer and burning indigestion, take Calc. Sulph. before a meal and chew a walnut-sized piece of raw peeled potato with it. If there is no appetite, which sometimes happens as we age, two Calc. Sulph. tablets sucked three times daily will help to restore enjoyment in food.

Calc. Sulph. is excellent for constipation as well as diarrhoea, and it is safe to take with other medications. Two Calc. Sulph. tablets should be sucked every 20–30 minutes until the diarrhoea stops. Calc. Fluor., Calc. Sulph., Nat. Mur., Nat. Sulph. and Silica work well together when people travel and are affected by different foods. In this situation, dissolve three tablets of each salt in hot water and sip 3–4 times through the day. This quick-and-easy hot tissue salt tea should be taken first thing in the morning and last thing at night, and even after the midday meal if necessary, to settle digestion. It is important to note that if a condition does not clear up within a day or two, a doctor should be consulted. The dosages here are general ones; if in doubt, do not delay in seeking medical support.

The diet

The persistent desire for salty foods or snacks, especially crisps washed down with iced cola (known as 'the cola-and-chips syndrome'), is common, even in the elderly. Two Calc. Sulph. tablets sucked 2–3 times daily will ease these cravings. Other food cravings, such as for chocolate or sweets, also indicate the need for Calc. Sulph.

The liver, bladder and kidneys

As we age, we tend to accumulate small health problems, which can become bigger if not addressed. Bladder and kidney complaints top the list, as well as 'liverishness', as my grandmother called being unwell and irritable, with aches and pains. Age spots or liver spots on the back of the hands, bladder aches, muscle aches and joint aches all indicate that Calc. Sulph. is in short supply. To remedy this, take two Mag. Phos. tablets with two Calc. Sulph. tablets 6–8 times a day for three days. This will counteract the aches and pains. Eat foods rich in Calc. Sulph. and add Silica as a secondary salt. Remember that the liver carries the burden in the body, and worn-out toxic cells can accumulate and overload it. Calc. Sulph. is needed urgently here, as it helps to clear out and repair. If you have taken painkillers such as aspirin or coal tar medication for any length of time, suck two Calc. Sulph. tablets frequently to clear the liver.

Sleep

The 'sleep formula' I learned early on in my work with tissue salts is easy to remember, as it includes all the phosphates: numbers 2, 4 6, 8 and 10. However, I have learned that Calc. Sulph. is an important addition, as it helps with restlessness.

As we age, a good night's sleep becomes rare, and I have become particularly grateful to the tissue salts for their assistance. The 'sleep formula' has been my lifesaver, especially when there is a full day of work ahead. The days can be tiring when you are older, and the desire for sleep comes early, but we often wake at midnight or in the small hours and lie thinking anxiously or filled with despair. Here is a way to manage this: put on a warm dressing gown and slippers, make a hot-water bottle and tuck some fresh lavender sprigs or rose-scented pelargonium leaves between the hot-water bottle and its cover. The fragrance is calming and unwinding, so keep a bowl of the sprigs on the kitchen table. You will come to rely on it in the middle of the night. It is so gently soothing! Make yourself hot milk or chamomile or melissa tea, add a touch of honey and crush 2–4 Calc. Sulph. tablets, 2–4 Calc. Phos. tablets and two Kali. Phos. tablets into the drink, and take it back to bed with you. I often say the comforting prayer I have come to rely on as I sip my warm, soothing drink!

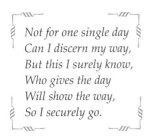

Not for one single day
Can I discern my way,
But this I surely know,
Who gives the day
Will show the way,
So I securely go.

How you feel

Calc. Sulph. is of great importance in 'pressing the start button' when there is fatigue, listlessness, inability to get started, and engulfing worries, often about imaginary problems. When we find ourselves unable to 'get up and go', and procrastination becomes very evident, we can be sure that we are short of Calc. Sulph. Two tablets sucked 3–6 times a day is the perfect remedy, and a bowl of good oats porridge with six almonds chopped in, a fresh or dried fig, and a few plums or prunes, will be a good start to the day, with a glass or two of barley water later in the day.

3 Calc. Sulph.

Secondary and complementary tissue salts

Mag. Phos. and Silica both work beautifully with Calc. Sulph., clearing chronic discharge anywhere in the body. Become familiar with Kali. Phos. too, as it fits in very well here, distributing oxygen and working on the third (chronic) level of infection . It can be added to the above formulas if needed.

Herbs that contain Calc. Sulph.

Asthma tree/Vasaka (*Adhotoda vasica*): I have included the extraordinary asthma tree here as it is rich in Calc. Fluor., is a natural bronchodilator and is one of the most useful herbs for chest and respiratory ailments, particularly in the aged. In cases of bronchitis, copious mucus and respiratory distress, take two cups of the leaf tea daily to obtain relief and comfort. To make the tea, pour a cup of boiling water over one or two leaves, with the bitter midrib removed. Add an avocado leaf if possible and crush it into the tea with a spoon (see more in *100 New Herbs*). We post cuttings of this pretty, easy-to-grow tree countrywide.

Red clover (*Trifolium pratense*): The amazing red clover is a shining star for Calc. Sulph. It is a diuretic, flushing out toxins, and is also rich in calcium and Silica. Enjoy it in a stir-fry as well as in salads, soups and stews. Pick fresh leaves daily, as in the heat of midsummer it can get mildew. If this is the case, cut back all the affected leaves and discard them in a bin or burn them (do not put them in the compost heap). As an antispasmodic, this precious plant can be made into a tea with ginger and honey to ease a thick phlegmy cough, relax tight breathing, and it will also act as a pain reliever. We post red clover seed countrywide as it is so vital as a health-boost tea and green food. Try growing it – you will love it!

Stinging nettle (*Urtica dioica*): This is the main cleansing and detoxifying herb; however, parsley and celery have a similar action and are also excellent. All are rich in Calc. Sulph. and serve to detoxify, cleanse, repair and restore. Arthritic conditions and gout benefit from their action, and rhinitis and hay fever lessen. To make a tea from any of these herbs, pour a cup of boiling water over ¼ cup fresh herb. Let the tea stand for five minutes, then stir well, strain and sip slowly with two Calc. Sulph. tablets. Their tonic and cleansing action in the blood takes us towards the vitality we all need!

Wormwood (*Artemesia absinthun*): This plant is rich in Calc. Sulph., but it is extremely bitter. *Artemesia Africa* (wilde als), our indigenous wormwood, also eases stomach pain and stimulates the secretion of bile. Rather use wormwood in a poultice to reduce swelling and infections. To make the poultice, pour eight cups of boiling water over two cups of fresh wilde als leaves and sprigs. Let it stand until it's warm, then stir well and dip a small towel into the brew. Place the poultice over the swollen area for 20 minutes, keeping it warm. The wormwoods and all *Artemesias* ɐ powerful and bitter and need very careful dosages. *Remember: when in doubt, leave out!*

Foods rich in Calc. Sulph.

Below is a list of vibrant and health-boosting foods filled with Calc. Sulph. and rich in vitamins, minerals and amino acids. We should grow them ourselves and eat at least eight daily!

Celery, parsley and fennel are wonderful in salads, soups, smoothies, juices and stir-fries, and delicious meals can be created around them. For natural antibiotics and superb clearing of chest and bladder infections, use onions, garlic, leeks and spring onions; they are easy to grow, so plant them in abundance! Radishes, watercress, asparagus, cauliflower, cucumber, wheatgrass, barley grass, oat grass, lentils and almonds all clear toxins and build vitality, flush the kidneys and boost the circulation, while figs and prunes help to ease constipation and to clear the kidneys and colon.

Old-fashioned barley water

Barley water is a treasure that is too often neglected. It lowers cholesterol, detoxifies, cleanses, fortifies and helps recuperation. Below is an old-fashioned yet wonderful recipe that should be part of our daily lives, especially given the anti-ageing benefits and vitality it brings.

Simmer a cup of pearl barley in two litres of water, using a heavy-bottomed pot. Keep the water level constant and top up if needed, as the water boils away easily. After 40 minutes, set the pot aside to cool, keeping it covered. Strain and serve the liquid chilled with a squeeze of fresh lemon juice, a slice of lemon (no sugar) and ice, and sip slowly. A glass a day will ensure that you thrive!

Calc. Sulph. broth

SERVES 4

As Calc. Sulph. is such a valuable cleanser and infection fighter, this wonderfully cleansing broth will become a year-round favourite, and it acts as an anti-inflammatory treatment too!

Olive oil
4–6 leeks, sliced thinly
2 medium-sized onions, sliced thinly
3–4 cups sliced radishes, green leaves included
1 small cauliflower, broken into florets and a few finely shredded
  outer leaves
10 fresh asparagus spears, sliced into 1cm-long pieces
2 cups chopped celery, green leaves included
2 cups thinly sliced fennel bulb
1 cup chopped fennel leaves
2 litres fresh chicken stock (made with chicken bones)
Himalayan salt to taste
Paprika to taste
Juice and zest of a lemon

Heat the olive oil in a large, heavy-bottomed pot and stir-fry the leeks and onions. Add the remaining ingredients and bring to the boil, topping up with more chicken stock or water if needed. The broth will be light, tasty and not at all like a heavy soup. You can add chopped fresh watercress and parsley when serving. Serve in big mugs with a spoon.

   This broth will give your immune system a boost and is a great recipe for treating the liver and kidneys, as well as for slimmers.

4 Ferrum Phos.

Iron Phosphate • *Ferrum Phosphoricum*

Consistent health begins with the right level of iron phosphate in the blood. It actually depends on it. In all my years of working with tissue salts I have never taken Ferrum Phos. for granted, as the tiny molecules of this tissue salt are connected chemically to the oxygen we inhale. They carry the oxygen to all parts of the body, which results in glowing health and vitality.

Should there be a deficiency of Ferrum Phos. in the blood, the body compensates by increasing the rate of circulation in order to carry sufficient oxygen to the extremities. The increased rate of blood flow leads to the body becoming warm and a 'fever' may be experienced, due primarily to lack of oxygen. This is a consequence of iron deficiency because iron is the oxygen carrier! Ferrum Phos. is able to strengthen the walls of the blood vessels and enhance their ability to distribute oxygen-rich blood to all the cells.

Ferrum Phos. is the biochemic 'first-aid salt', essential to health and life, and for this reason it should be taken frequently when there is evident lack. In later life we need Ferrum Phos. daily to increase the health of the entire circulatory system. I often suggest this, especially when I see lack of energy and vitality and a flushed face and bloodshot eyes. Two Ferrum Phos. tablets will ease a feeling of faintness quickly, and if sucked every 15–20 minutes for the next 3–4 hours, they often change the outcome completely! It is a true first-aid tissue salt. I often suggest to the elderly that they keep Ferrum Phos. and Mag. Phos. next to the bed!

The head

Vertigo, dizziness, headache that can cause temporary blindness in an eye, a rush of blood to the head when bending, as well as confusion, upset, agitation, incoherence and a flushed face and head sore to the touch, all call for Ferrum Phos. If the head is sore to the touch, there may also be sores and inflammation on the scalp. Equilibrium can be restored within an hour by sucking two Ferrum Phos. tablets every 10 minutes.

4 Ferrum Phos.

The eyes

Ferrum Phos. is needed when the eyes are sore, red and watery, when it is painful to move the eyes from one object to another, and when the eyes feel dry and sandpapery. The first stages of retinitis can be eased quickly by sucking two Ferrum Phos. tablets every 20 minutes until the eyes feel soothed.

The ears

Throbbing earache, perhaps with a cold or after a cold has cleared up, and where there is temporary deafness, sharp pains and noises in the ears like water roaring, all indicate a 'disequilibrium' of the blood vessels and lack of Ferrum Phos. There may also be redness and soreness of the outer ear, again indicating lack of Ferrum Phos. Suck two tablets every 10 minutes until symptoms ease.

The nose

When there is a nose bleed without an injury or the first signs of a cold coming on, either a pale face or a flushed high temperature, or catarrhal feverishness with a blocked nose, suck Calc. Phos., Kali. Phos. and Nat. Sulph. with Ferrum Phos. (two tablets of each) every 15–30 minutes until the symptoms ease.

Oral health

Hot swollen gums, mouth ulcers, fever blisters, gum infections and a predisposition to bleeding gums indicate that Ferrum Phos. is in short supply. Suck two tablets at least six times a day, allowing the tablets to dissolve slowly in the mouth.

In the case of inflammatory conditions of the gums, and toothache, use Ferrum Phos. and Mag. Phos. to ease the pain until you can get to a dentist. When there is a red inflamed tongue, suck two Ferrum Phos. tablets frequently; allow the tablets to dissolve in the mouth and hold them as long as possible on the tongue before swallowing.

The tissue salts we have made for us are lactose-free, and literally soften in the mouth. This is what Dr Schuessler wanted, for in this way the tissue salts enter the bloodstream directly via the soft mucous membranes of the mouth.

For sore throats, dry inflamed throat ulcers, and late-onset chickenpox where pustules form down the throat, crush and dissolve 10 Ferrum Phos. tablets in a glass of hot water, as hot as is comfortable, and take frequent sips. Hold the fluid in the mouth and let it trickle gently down the throat. Do this every half hour or so until the symptoms ease.

Early writings on tissue salts recommended Ferrum Phos. with Calc. Sulph. and Kali. Mur. for quinsy (peritonsillar abscess) and inflammation of the tonsils, and I have found this trio to be excellent. When diphtheria was prevalent, these three tissue salts were the accepted treatment under medical supervision, taken every 30 minutes until there was a feeling of relief. Interestingly, they also work beautifully together for singers and public speakers as they strengthen the voice. Remember these three tissue salts when the voice sounds croaky and uneven.

The circulatory system

When there are heart palpitations or a rapid pulse, such as with fevers and anaemia for example, or when there is high blood pressure, take two tablets each of Ferrum Phos. and Kali. Phos. every 10 minutes, then every 30 minutes. Lessen the dose as the condition eases, until you can get to a doctor. This will bring a great deal of relief, but whenever there is doubt and anxiety, do not try to treat yourself. Abide by your doctor's decisions and stay in touch with him or her. Add these two superb salts to the daily medications and feel the difference – they are very comforting!

The digestive system

When there is colic after eating, or nausea, vomiting and diarrhoea of undigested foods, or if there is a tendency towards digestive upsets, especially as we age, suck two Ferrum Phos. and two Mag. Phos. tablets every 15 minutes, or dissolve 10 tablets each of Mag. Phos. and Ferrum Phos. into a glass of hot water and sip it before, during or after a meal. The condition will soon clear.

Calc. Phos. and Ferrum Phos. make an excellent combination for heart-burn, burping, flatulence and even constipation. However, do not forget the comfort of an old-fashioned hot-water bottle held over the abdomen. I tuck fresh lavender sprigs between the cover and the hot-water bottle, which promotes relaxation and eases the tension, especially if there is pain.

Where there is diarrhoea or more serious infections such as peritonitis, enteric fever, chronic diarrhoea and stools that are watery or contain undigested food, see your doctor immediately. Remember that tissue salts can be taken safely alongside any pharmaceutical medications. Bleeding haemorrhoids also respond to Ferrum Phos. and Calc. Fluor. I make a comforting cream for this that is very soothing when applied frequently.

Haemorrhoid cream

1 cup pennywort leaves (*Centella asiatica*)
½ cup yarrow leaves (*Achillea millefolium*)
1 cup good aqueous cream
10 Ferrum Phos. tablets
4 tablets each of Calc. Fluor., Calc. Phos., Kali. Mur., Kali. Sulph.,
   Nat. Mur. and Silica
2 tablespoons hot water
2 teaspoons vitamin E oil
4 teaspoons olive oil

Simmer the pennywort, yarrow and aqueous cream in a double boiler (see *My 100 Favourite Herbs* for more information on these herbs). Stir frequently and press the herbs against the sides of the pot to release the healing oils. Simmer for 20 minutes. Set the mixture aside to cool for 20 minutes. Strain through a new sieve that has been sterilised and discard the leaves. Mix in the tissue salts, dissolved together in the hot water, and add the vitamin E oil and olive oil. Stir the cream thoroughly. Spoon into sterilised glass jars with good lids and label. Apply the cream generously and frequently to the haemorrhoids.

The urinary system

At the first twinge of cystitis, reach for Ferrum Phos.! Suck two tablets each of Ferrum Phos. and Nat. Phos. every 15–20 minutes, then take the tablets every 30 minutes over a two-hour period, and then take them hourly. A severe attack can often be averted in this way. Once the acute phase is over, take two tablets of each every 2–3 hours through the day.

The same formula will help with burning after urination, and urinary incontinence from a weak sphincter muscle. As a physiotherapist I taught women of all ages, particularly menopausal and elderly women, how to tighten the pelvic floor muscles: Cross the legs, press ankles and knees together while standing or lying down, and pull up the pelvic floor muscles as strongly as possible; hold your breath and then release. Repeat this at least 10 times when you get a chance. In this way the urethral sphincter and bladder are strengthened. In the elderly, wetting the bed due to weak muscles is distressing, so become aware of the importance of this easy exercise to strengthen the neck of the bladder and the pelvic floor.

Kali. Phos. with Ferrum Phos. helps here too; suck two tablets about six times a day. When there is a constant urge to urinate, Kali. Phos., Nat. Mur. and Ferrum Phos. is a comforting formula (two tablets of each 6–10 times through the day). Remember that a hot drink, especially before bedtime, also helps: dissolve six Ferrum Phos., six Nat. Mur. and six Kali. Phos. tablets in half a glass of hot water and sip slowly. This formula also helps if there is any inflammation in the kidneys.

Female problems
Irregular menstruation and excessive bleeding are eased with Ferrum Phos. Suck two tablets frequently and add Mag. Phos. if there are cramps. In the case of menopause, if there are hot flushes, vertigo, fluid retention, a florid complexion, distress, anxiety and a feeling of helplessness, suck two tablets each of Ferrum Phos. and Kali. Phos. every 15–20 minutes until you feel better. This will soothe things reliably. Because of my work with tissue salts, I sailed through menopause and was hardly aware of it. Be reassured that tissue salts work and that 'this too shall pass'!

How you feel
When Ferrum Phos. is included daily, problems lighten and resolve themselves. In the case of forgetfulness, irritability, depression, fatigue, panic attacks, and feeling overheated and desperate, remember my personal uplifter: two tablets each of Calc. Phos., Ferrum Phos. and Kali. Phos. sucked slowly and quietly. Or make a hot 'rescue' drink by dissolving four tablets of each in a cup of hot water (boil the water, then cool it to a pleasant temperature) and sip slowly. This is a little lifesaver that will even soothe a crisis. I have come to rely on it for a host of problems and am always grateful for its efficacy.

Secondary and complementary tissue salts
Kali. Mur. works exceptionally well with Ferrum Phos. to soothe the inflammatory processes and stimulate the immune system. These two tissue salts also work together wonderfully to normalise congested mucous membranes, heart palpitations, excessive bleeding and shortness of breath.

Kali. Sulph. works well with Ferrum Phos. to improve oxygenation of the tissues. When there is a tight cough with loss of breath, dissolve four tablets each of Ferrum Phos. and Kali. Sulph. in a cup of hot water and sip slowly. Similarly, when a little food 'goes down the wrong way', the cough can be alleviated by sipping a hot drink of Kali. Sulph. and Ferrum Phos. or by sucking two tablets of each carefully so as not to choke!

In the case of anaemia, make a hot drink with four Ferrum Phos. and four Nat. Mur. tablets and sip a cup or two a day. An excellent treatment when there are hot, sore, swollen joints is four tablets each of Ferrum Phos., Nat. Mur. and Nat. Phos in a cup of hot water.

Other ailments

On days when you feel you are not managing, and backache, pains over the kidneys, stiffness and rheumatism take a toll, Ferrum Phos. is a panacea. Suck two tablets frequently and add a little Silica, especially for the hip joints and lower back pain and when there are feelings of helplessness. For strains, sprains, varicose veins and general pain immobility, reach for the Ferrum Phos.

Ancient texts on the wonders of tissue salts all recommended Calc. Fluor. alternating with Ferrum Phos. for bone fractures, hip joint fractures, rheumatic lameness, threatened aneurism, phlebitis, palpitations of the heart and epilepsy, and all recorded excellent results!

Reddened complexion, nose bleeds, fevers and swellings respond to Ferrum Phos. as it relaxes, eases and calms. Sleeplessness can create despair, but all the phosphate tissue salts, from Calc. Phos. to Nat. Phos., will ease the situation. Increase Ferrum Phos. and reduce sugar, as it compromises the immune system, and you will feel better for it.

Shortness of breath after a brisk walk, or after any exertion, can be eased by sucking two Ferrum Phos. tablets, which makes exercising so much easier. This is an important tissue salt to keep the body fit and strong – do not neglect it.

Herbs that contain Ferrum Phos.

Celery (*Apium graveolens*): Celery is nature's diuretic and urinary antiseptic, and has antispasmodic properties. It also improves the circulation, reduces pain and lowers high blood pressure.

Dandelion (*Taraxacum officinale*): As dandelion is rich in iron, I try to include a few leaves in my daily salad. I bought seeds of a luscious and prolific dandelion from Kew Gardens in England many years ago, which is not the same as the international dandelions we find growing as weeds in our lawns. It is one is the best ones to eat, and three chopped dandelion leaves in a salad of celery, avocado, lettuce, rocket, buckwheat leaves and flowers, moistened with a squeeze of lemon juice, is absolutely delicious – it's a combination I never grow tired of!

Horseradish (*Armoracia rusticana*): This herb is well worth growing, as it is good for circulation, eases coughs, colds, chest ailments, sore muslces, strains and sprains, and is excellent for arthritis sufferers, as it helps to lubricate stiff joints.

Parsley (*Petroselinum crispum*): This herb is a superb cleaner and tonic. Try to eat two or three sprigs every day. It is also a natural diuretic and eases cystitis, delayed menstruation, liverishness and prostate pain.

Foods rich in Ferrum Phos.

Fresh fruit, vegetables and herbs rich in Ferrum Phos. are a natural remedy for all the ailments listed above and need to form part of our daily diet. Grow your own salads year-round to flush toxins, clear infections, to keep the bladder and kidneys fit and the prostate working well, and feel how good your energy levels are. It all begins with a daily salad platter! Include radishes, spring onions, baby spinach, sesame seeds, walnuts and lemon juice, and pile on a selection of sprouts. I call this 'the anti-ageing salad'!

Oat straw tea

4 cups oat straw, cut into short lengths
2 litres water
3 thumb-length sprigs fresh stinging nettle
3 pennywort leaves

Simmer the oat straw in water in a heavy-bottomed pot for 30 minutes. To make the tea really potent I add stinging nettle and pennywort leaves. Allow the brew to cool to a comfortable warmth, strain and keep it in the fridge, covered. Each time you need a cup (try for two cups a day), pour it from the jug and warm it to a pleasant temperature, or add it to chilled berry juice. I whirl a cup of fresh berries (blackberries or silver cane berries are best) in the liquidiser with a touch of honey and a cup of oat straw tea, and then dilute with another cup of the tea and drink it with a squeeze of lemon and some ice on a hot day.

Lean grilled meat salad

SERVES 4

2 cups brown lentils
Juice of 1 lemon
Himalayan salt to taste
12 thin slices lean beef
olive oil
2 medium onions, peeled and cut into thick slices
1 butter lettuce
6–10 baby potatoes, boiled and cooled
½ cup chopped parsley
½ cup sesame seeds
1 cup sliced radishes

Dressing
½ cup olive oil
½ cup horseradish sauce
½ cup lemon juice
½ cup honey

Cook the lentils in water, drain and allow them to cool, then toss with lemon juice and season with salt. Brush the beef with olive oil and lemon juice and season with salt. Grill the beef slices and the onion slices. To assemble, put lettuce leaves in a bowl, add the lentils, potatoes, onion, radish and beef slices. Sprinkle with parsley and sesame seeds.

To make the dressing, pour the ingredients into a screw-top glass jar and shake it well. Pour over the salad just before serving.

If you are taking this salad to work, keep the sauce in a separate bottle and pour on the salad just before eating to prevent it becoming soggy.

Foods rich in Ferrum Phos. include all varieties of spinach (including the prolific and easy-to-grow New Zealand spinach which has deliciously tender leaves for salads, soups and stir-fries), lentils (grow your own and grow lentil sprouts), radishes, onions, spring onions, leeks and Welsh onions. Lettuce and all varieties of garlic are rich in iron. Try growing your own garlic and chop a delicious young plant, leaves included, into your salad!

Lean red meat and liver are another excellent source of iron. The meat should be raised without steroids and hormones and grilled with lemon juice. Almonds, walnuts and sesame seeds are also rich in Ferrum Phos. and healthy stir-fries, soups and stews are the most important foods to build health. Include chickpeas, green beans, broad beans, brown rice and tomatoes (grow your own cherry tomatoes throughout spring, summer and autumn) and harvest the summer bounty for winter soups and stews. Oats and oats straw are rich in Ferrum Phos. Grow your own and dry the oats for teas to ease aching joints and backs, and to treat osteoporosis.

Making horseradish sauce

Horseradish becomes dormant in winter, and this is the time when it is ready for digging up.

Wash the rhizomes well, scrubbing off the dirt. Then peel the horseradish with a potato peeler, wearing goggles to protect your eyes and a mask over your mouth, as it is far worse than onions and makes your eyes water considerably.

Push the roots through a grinder, then spoon the minced horseradish into a screw-top glass bottle. Heat 2 cups of white grape vinegar and 1½ cups of caramel sugar in a pot and allow the sugar to dissolve. Stir in 3 teaspoons of crushed coriander seeds. Spoon the mixture into the bottle with the horseradish. Seal and label. Serve with roast beef or spread onto toast with Cheddar cheese.

5 _Kali. Mur._

Potassium Chloride • Chloride of Potash •
Kalium Muriaticum

Kali. Mur. is vitally important in building fibrin, a fibrous protein involved in blood clotting. Brain cells cannot form without fibrin, nor can nerves, muscles or blood. Kali. Mur. is therefore an exceptional tissue salt for protecting, clearing and sustaining good health, and it works beautifully with Kali. Sulph. which is a cell oxygenator.

Kali. Mur. is also a natural decongestant and a lymph and blood conditioner, and its role in clearing skin ailments and debilitating congestions in the ears, nose and throat gives it star status in my book!

In my many years of researching tissue salts I have remained grateful to Kali. Mur. for its role in relieving distressing ailments such as croup, cystitis, boils and eczema. I have made a long list of its specific healing abilities, and I have noticed how organically grown herbs and foods that contain Kali. Mur. relieve these conditions. Something I learned from a pathologist is that all the conditions listed below are exacerbated by carbonated drinks.

This is a marvellous tissue salt for the ageing yet active citizen. Aches and pains, stuffy nose, blocked ears, deafness, heavy moods, and even grief and despair are relieved. I have come to rely on Kali. Mur. increasingly and value its reliability, especially when irritability and worries occur. Try a cup of Kali. Mur. tea made with ginger and basil, as it is very comforting after a stressful day.

The skeleton and joints

Older people can experience random aches such as backache, shoulder pains, neck pains, joint pains, stiffness, dull aches and lack of mobility; even stretching or lying down can bring discomfort. Kali. Mur., Mag. Phos., Ferrum Phos. and Nat. Phos. make a comforting and soothing formula that will ease this discomfort. Dissolve 4–8 tablets of each in a cup of hot water and sip frequently. Here is where exercise, such as walking, and a diet rich in fruit, vegetables and stevia (fresh or dried leaves, not the white powder) will begin to change the entire system. Walk every day, extending the distance little by little, especially if you spend a lot of time sitting.

The head, scalp and hair

When there is a headache, check the tongue; if there is a thick white coating this will indicate that the liver is affected due to lack of bile, often with constipation and a bloated feeling, while a sickly headache with nausea can occur after eating rich food. Suck two Kali. Mur. tablets every 10 minutes until you feel relief, or make a Kali. Mur. and Nat. Sulph. drink with 6–10 tablets of each dissolved in a cup of hot water (I always boil the water first in a stainless steel kettle – not a plastic one – and then allow it to cool to a comfortable heat). Sip slowly. The diet becomes important in these cases and there will be a positive response to increased Kali. Mur. intake, plus you will feel a lift in spirit too.

White, flaky dandruff on the scalp shows the need for Kali. Mur. Take it daily for this ailment. It is a valuable scalp treatment and can be made into a final rinse for use after shampooing. Dissolve 10–20 Kali. Mur. tablets in a litre of hot water. Use this, diluted with another litre of cold water to make the final temperature comfortable, and massage into the scalp thoroughly. It can also be dabbed onto the scalp to clear dandruff. The rinse keeps well; just stir it each time before applying. Kali. Mur. is also excellent for thinning fragile hair, so take two tablets morning and evening. It seems to give new vitality to the hair, and combined with borage in the hair rinse below, it is excellent. You will find that your hair and scalp respond beautifully!

Borage hair rinse

3 cups borage leaves, stems and flowers
2 litres water
20 Kali. Mur. tablets, finely crushed

Simmer the borage and water in a stainless steel pot for 30 minutes with the lid on. Set the mixture aside to cool, then strain. Dissolve the Kali. Mur. tablets in the brew and use as a rinse after shampooing or apply to the scalp on soaked cotton wool pads. After a couple of weeks the dry, flaky scalp will disappear. In addition, take 6–8 Kali. Mur. tablets morning and evening, crushed in a hot drink, or suck two tablets 4–6 times every day.

5 Kali. Mur.

Eyes, ears, nose and throat

Kali. Mur. decongests and aids recovery quite rapidly. Any crusts or mucus discharge and build-up in the corners of the eyes call for Kali. Mur. Suck two tablets frequently and make a lotion to wipe the eyes and nose.

Thick mucus with a blocked nose and sinuses, and a phlegmy throat and chest, can make one miserable. Blocked ears, buzzing sounds, and swollen tonsils and adenoids all indicate that Kali. Mur. is needed. Suck two tablets every 15–20 minutes until relief is found. Where there are swollen neck lymph glands, eye discharge and nasal catarrh, Kali. Mur. comes to the rescue. Remember that it is part of the comforting flu formula (tissue salts 1, 4, 5, 9 and 11).

The two best tissue salts for colds and a runny nose, sinusitis and clear runny mucus are Kali. Mur. and Ferrum Phos. In the prolific sneezing, wheezing and coughing stages of infection, sucking two tablets of each frequently will ease all symptoms, including watery eyes and blocked ears. Ferrum Phos. should be taken alternately with Kali. Mur. during hay fever attacks to compensate for the outflow of fibrin (in the mucus being expelled). This will ease the sneezing, coughing and general distress.

For ear infections with fluid and pressure in the ear, and post-infection when hearing is affected, take two Kali. Mur. tablets frequently. Do the same when the ear canal feels clogged and the Eustachian tube is blocked and no amount of nose-blowing, yawning or swallowing relieves this. Kali. Mur. helps to keep the canals open and hearing clear. Suck two tablets frequently during air travel to keep the ears from blocking and buzzing.

Oral health

For thrush in the mouth and a thick, slimy feeling in the throat, dissolve 10 crushed Kali. Mur. tablets in water to make a gargle; sip slowly and gargle in the mouth before swallowing. This will quickly ease the discomfort.

Taking tissue salts

Tissue salts are designed to dissolve quickly in the mouth so that the minute particles can go to work immediately through the mucous membrane, and from there into the fine capillaries and the bloodstream. This is why tissue salts work so effectively. Dissolved in hot water and held in the mouth for a few seconds before swallowing, they effectively set healing in motion.

The respiratory system

Kali. Mur. is absolutely essential for a croupy cough, tight chest, asthma, pleurisy and even pneumonia. Suck two Kali. Mur. tablets frequently with all the other flu remedy tissue salts (numbers 1, 4, 5, 9 and 11).

Croup-like hoarseness in a cough indicates that Kali. Mur. is deficient and that pleurisy may arise (add Kali. Phos. for easier breathing). Whooping cough can apparently occur at any age, producing an abundance of white phlegm. Suck two Kali. Mur. tablets frequently until relief is found.

The digestive system

Kali. Mur. plays a role in the production of saliva, which is actually the first stage of digestion. It also establishes a good rhythm in the digestive system, and sour belching, flatulence, bloating, discomfort, and burning sensations in the stomach and bowel are dispersed merely by sucking two Kali. Mur. tablets frequently. A cup of peppermint tea will aid this.

Peppermint Kali. Mur. tea for digestion

1 thumb-length piece of fresh peppermint
1 cup of boiling water
4–6 Kali. Mur. tablets

Pour the boiling water over the peppermint and allow it to stand for five minutes. Stir it well, and dissolve the tissue salts in the brew. Sip the tea hot, holding it in the mouth before swallowing.

Remember that too much sugar and too many refined or fatty foods and carbonated drinks clog the gut and tax the liver, and are the very things that age us. Make your own healthy cool-drinks, teas and treats using dates, grapes, raisins and apple juice. Life is precious and you need to be fit, strong and well in the golden years.

Kali. Mur. actually thins the blood, which is why it is so important for the liver. Broths and cleansing vegetable soups are valuable to keep the liver functioning well and when made with foods rich in Kali. Mur., they form a good base from which to work. As we get older, liver congestion becomes a frequent reality, and fried and fatty foods, and too many

5 Kali. Mur.

artificial flavourings, overload it mercilessly. This liver congestion is ageing to the whole body. Liver health should be a primary concern.

My liver detox broth is a healthy and surprisingly tasty light soup that can be served in a mug as a liver cleanser, and it is quick and easy to make. Flavoured with celery, paprika or red pepper, lemon juice and a small amount of salt, it is a wonderful snack at any time of the day and goes to work on the liver quickly. I call it Kali. Mur. cleanse.

The circulatory system

Kali. Mur. eases the heart palpitations that can occur as a result of intense stress and anxiety. In their books, doctors Carey and Perry recommend a daily dose of Kali. Mur., morning and evening, for heart ailments. A cough with palpitations can also be soothed with Kali. Mur. Dissolve 10 tablets in a cup of boiling water and sip it slowly as a hot drink; it will soon steady and calm you. However, always consult and follow the advice of a medical practitioner if you have any heart problems or irregularities.

Female problems

To ease menstrual pain, postmenopausal discomfort and bloating, and congested haemorrhoids, dissolve 4–8 tablets each of Kali. Mur., Ferrum Phos., Nat. Mur. and Nat. Phos. in a cup of hot water and sip slowly. It will do wonders for women who struggle with postmenopause symptoms or hot flushes.

When there is thick, white mucous discharge known as leucorrhoea, or in cases of cystitis, vaginitis and even cystic fibrosis, Kali. Mur. and Ferrum Phos. are essential. Take two tablets of each 4–8 times through the day. Persist with this little formula as it is very comforting and will also help with accompanying cramps and dull pains in the abdomen. Also, examine your diet and opt for light broths, soups and steamed vegetables to replace heavy meat and fried foods.

Male problems

The prostate gland responds well to Kali. Mur., and when there is swelling of the testicles and spongy enlargement (often with dark-coloured urine), suck two Kali. Mur. tablets up to 10 times through the day, and dissolve 10 Ferrum Phos. and 10 Kali. Mur. tablets in a cup of boiling water and sip frequently. Also, check your diet, avoid sugar and fried foods, and rather eat home-made broths and vegetable soups.

Kali. Mur. cleanse (detox broth)

SERVES 4–6

1 cup chopped onions, green leaves included
2 tablespoons olive oil
1 cup finely grated carrots
1 cup finely chopped celery
1 cup finely chopped borage
1 cup finely chopped fennel
1 cup finely chopped kale
1 cup finely chopped basil
1 cup finely grated squash
1 cup brown lentils or lentil sprouts
Juice of 1 lemon
1 tablespoon finely grated ginger
1–2 teaspoons Himalayan salt crystals
Paprika or red pepper to taste
2 litres water

Brown the onions in the olive oil. Add all the other ingredients and simmer for 40 minutes or until the vegetables are soft. Adjust the seasoning, sprinkle fresh chopped parsley on top with a slice of lemon, and serve the broth hot. I find that fresh fennel and paprika or red pepper give it a wonderful taste. The soup can also be whirled in a blender to make a delicious late-afternoon snack on a cold day, giving you vitality and clearing up a cold quickly.

The skin

Kali. Mur. is excellent for weeping eczema, rashes, crusty exudations, eruptions, powdery scale, acne, pustules, pimples, small festering sores, inflamed weeping scratches, and grazes. It is also good for shingles, as well as the itchy soreness of chilblains in winter. Surprisingly, Kali. Mur. is the main tissue salt for lupus. Suck two tablets at least 4–8 times through the day. In the case of burns, sunburn, chafed skin and blisters, suck two tablets each of Kali. Mur. and Ferrum Phos. frequently. A lotion can be made by dissolving 10 tablets of each in a cup of hot water. Let the lotion cool and then spray it on the skin for soothing relief.

5 | Kali. Mur.

Other ailments

Kali. Mur. is a valuable tissue salt, as it helps relieve many familiar ailments: liver problems including jaundice, toxicity, overloaded liver, cirrhosis and hepatitis; feelings of weariness and heaviness; respiratory problems; itchy blisters and crusts on the scalp; glandular fever; ongoing inflammation of the hip or elbow joint; candida; psoriasis and itchy skin; and white ulcers in the mouth. All respond to Kali. Mur. – suck two tablets frequently or dissolve 6–8 Kali. Mur. tablets in a glass of hot water and sip it slowly.

How you feel

Kali. Mur. is of benefit when one is unable to 'let go' of upsetting incidents, and when there is rehashing of past hurts and events that caused upset. Remember that Kali. Mur. is a 'waste disposer'; it helps us to get over past hurts, to 'spit it all out', literally, and to move on!

Secondary and complementary tissue salts

Ferrum Phos. is an excellent 'assistant' to Kali. Mur. in tackling immune dysfunction and restoring strength and vitality, particularly as we age. Together they clear away old problems including long-term discomfort, negative feelings, old coughs and mucus rumbling in the chest.

After Ferrum Phos. take Kali. Sulph. with Kali. Mur. to get rid of any old infections that have lingered too long, and every now and then give yourself a couple of days on Combin 12 (the combination of all 12 tissue salts in one tablet). Old niggles that have been neglected can be erased after 3–5 days of Ferrum Phos., Kali. Mur. and Kali. Sulph. followed by two Combin 12 tablets at least six times daily for a few days.

Herbs that contain Kali. Mur.

As you get to know and grow the Kali. Mur. herbs you will understand how marvellous they are and how perfectly they fit a pattern! For more information on these herbs, see *My 100 Favourite Herbs*.

Basil (*Ocimum* species): Perennial 'High Hopes Basil', 'Sacred Basil' and the annual basils are all excellent sources of Kali. Mur. and are valuable for their detoxifying, antiseptic, expectorant and even anti-depressant properties. I use basil fresh and finely chopped in salads, stir-fries, soups and stews, often mixed with chopped fresh parsley, as the minerals in both herbs are so bountiful. Basil also soothes itchy skin irritations, so I always have some growing close at hand!

Borage (*Borago officinalis*): Borage is also rich in Kali. Mur. and is known to ease eczema and skin irritations, as well as being a good expectorant and a strong antirheumatic herb and kidney tonic. Its blue flowers and leaves make a soothing and remarkable tea, and it is also healing in a soup, particularly for chest infections.

Fennel (*Foeniculum vulgare*): This herb is a good cleanser, detoxifier, diuretic and circulatory stimulant, as well as an anti-inflammatory and a mild yet comforting expectorant. I call it 'the slimmer's herb' as it helps to relieve fluid retention and bloating. It also eases stiffness in the muscles and flushes the kidneys, and it makes a fabulous drink, hot or cold, at any time of the day.

Ginger (*Zingiber officinalis*): This is a superb respiratory herb as it is a strong expectorant and promotes sweating to bring down a fever. Ginger also relaxes the peripheral blood vessels to enable waste products such as mucus to be removed, and it eases coughing and a sore throat. It can be taken in the form of a tea. To make it, pour a cup of boiling water over 4–6 thin slices of fresh root. Press the slices down well and stir with a teaspoon to release the juices. Add a teaspoon of honey and sip slowly. I find that chewing a sliver of the ginger root in the tea helps a persistent cough. The tea also eases nausea, colic, digestive stress and tight breathing. Both honey and ginger are antiseptic and therefore make an excellent treatment for a fever, tight chest and a clogged feeling in the nose and bronchi.

Mullein (*Verbascum thapsus*): This stately and showy biennial is excellent for clearing catarrh, mucus build-up and blocked Eustachian tubes, and it eases bronchitis, asthma and pneumonia. It also acts as an excellent expectorant, anti-inflammatory and wound cleanser. Make a tea from the leaves and flowers two or three times a day and sip slowly.

Sage (*Salvia officinalis*): One of the valuable natural antiseptics and antibiotics, sage promotes the flow of bile, lowers blood sugar levels, is a gentle yet reliable antispasmodic, and is excellent for respiratory problems. Often a cup of sage tea will steady us, calm a sneezing fit and ease a sore throat or cough. Together with honey and a good squeeze of lemon juice, it will relieve a cough and streaming cold and reduce the aches and pains of flu. It is so worth growing sage for this comfort! Have two cups a day if you can.

Violet (*Viola odorata*): I am particularly fond of violet tea to clear hay fever, a blocked nose, mucous cough, sinus build-up and headaches, especially those that are present upon waking. The flowers and leaves are edible, and the leaves can be used to make a pleasant tea. Violet is far more potent and useful than people realise. **NB: Do not use the African Violet (*Saintpaulia* species), as it is poisonous.**

Foods rich in Kali. Mur.

This is a wonderful list and many delicious dishes can be made from the following Kali. Mur.-rich foods: beetroot and beetroot leaves, green beans, carrots, squash, cucumbers, cauliflower, kale, asparagus, celery, mealies and mealie silk (grow your own non-genetically modified mealies), spinach, lentils, sesame seeds, and peaches, pineapples, apricots and lemons. Try to eat at least eight of these fruit and vegetables a day.

Kali. Mur. salad

SERVES 6–8

This has become a favourite salad at the Herbal Centre restaurant.

2 cups grated carrot
2 cups grated beetroot
2 cups thinly sliced cucumber
2–4 cups thinly shredded beetroot leaves
2 cups grated courgette squash
2 cups cooked green beans, chopped
2 cups chopped celery
2 cups young kale leaves, thinly shredded
2 cups chopped pineapple
2 cups chopped yellow peaches

Mix the ingredients together and dress with fresh lemon juice. With the addition of an avocado, this becomes a gourmet health salad, and with cooked broad beans or big butter beans, it is an almost perfect meal!

Asparagus for supper

Grow this wonderfully easy and exceptionally health-filled vegetable in the garden in rich, organic compost, edged with other food plants, such as parsley and celery. It is nothing short of spectacular and a single plant grows into a crown that pushes up those succulent spears during spring. In summer it has a froth of pretty fern-like fronds that carry seed capsules of brilliant orange.

Asparagus is a most effective kidney and bladder cleanser that helps to rid the body of accumulated toxins. There is no other plant quite as extraordinary in its detoxifying cleansing action as asparagus.

Pick the spears (10–12 per person) and boil them quickly until tender and serve with butter, lemon juice and a grinding of Himalayan salt. Rich in many vitamins and minerals, asparagus contains lots of Kali. Mur. as well as several other tissue salts. This is a remarkable health food!

6 _Kali. Phos._

Potassium Phosphate • _Kalium Phosphoricum_

This is an exceptional tissue salt as it helps to create a feeling of wellbeing by calming, quietening and steadying. Two Kali. Phos. tablets sucked slowly, while breathing deeply, will ease tension, anxiety, grief, fear and even misery. I have found Kali. Phos. to be vital in times of despair as well as during times of jangled nerves, helplessness and hypersensitivity.

In a person with a negative outlook, it is a builder of positivity. As such, it is as vital for the child as it is for the ageing grandparent and for everyone else in between! Kali. Phos. is essential to the elderly as it has the power to restore equilibrium, positivity and the will and desire to carry on.

When we have a confused and agitated outlook and are unable to make decisions, it means that Kali. Phos. is in short supply. Nervous disorders, including pessimism, irritability and over-reaction to trivial matters, can all be attributed to a lack of Kali. Phos. This can be corrected simply by taking more Kali. Phos. throughout the day. Kali. Phos. also has an antiseptic action, and of all the tissue salts it is unique in slowing down and repairing tissue decay and actually stopping the process of decay.

Dr Schuessler called it a 'balancing salt'. Where there is pain, discomfort and lack of healing in any area of the body, Kali. Phos. will regulate and correct the deficiency. For the body to thrive there must be a balance of nutritious food, daily exercise, daily elimination of waste products, and healthy blood containing all the elements necessary to build new cells. This balance depends on the amount of Kali. Phos. in the body. As we age, so each one of us will become more aware of that balance and the need to correct it.

For example, through over-eating or eating the wrong foods, the digestive system becomes clogged and uncomfortable and the results are colic, flatulence, irritable bowels and discomfort. However, this unhappy state of indigestion can be corrected with small doses of Kali. Phos. and with introduction of the super foods, which are particularly rich in Kali. Phos.

Kali. Phos. is a panacea we all need, and one of the safest 'medications' known to humankind. Let us not neglect it at any stage in our lives, but especially during the challenging ageing years. I look on Kali. Phos. as my 'rescue remedy' and keep it close at hand!

The head

When worry, confusion and a sickly headache cause us to falter, I have found my most comforting quick pick-up is a glass of hot water (boiled, then cooled to comfortable warmth) with 10 Kali. Phos., six Calc. Phos. and 10 Ferrum Phos. tablets dissolved in it and sipped slowly. It slows the panic, the pounding headache and confusion. Panic attacks are real and frightening, and you need to see your doctor about them. Depression is often diagnosed, even in those who seem to be coping. Healthy eating is the cornerstone to healing, as fast foods, chips, coffee, confectionery and processed food will worsen the condition and increase headaches. So be aware of what you eat.

Brain fatigue from overwork, and fretfulness, temper tantrums, crying, blaming others, poor memory, sensitivity to noise, mental confusion, nervousness, dizziness and a feeling that the head is swimming, all require Kali. Phos. Suck two tablets every 10 minutes for at least an hour or two.

The eyes

Dilated pupils, staring, looking startled, blurred and weakened vision, sleepwalking with eyes open and distorted vision will respond to Kali. Phos. Suck two tablets frequently, and where there is pain over the eyes or a facial neuralgia, include two Mag. Phos. tablets as well.

Bell's palsy is a sudden inflammation of the facial nerves causing a temporary paralysis on one side of the face; often the eye on the affected side cannot close. In these cases Kali. Phos. should be sucked every half hour for 3–4 hours, then every hour for 10–12 hours, and thereafter 4–6 times a day. This will gradually repair the facial paralysis; however, keep taking the medication from your doctor too.

Eye fatigue from staring at the computer screen for too long also can be alleviated with Kali. Phos. Suck two tablets slowly and frequently drink 10 tablets each of Kali. Phos. and Mag. Phos., dissolved in a glass of hot water.

Soothe eyes suffering from astigmatism, glaucoma, dryness, unfocused vision and fatigue with a warm Kali. Phos. compress. Dissolve 10 tablets each of Kali. Phos., Mag. Phos. and Ferrum Phos. in a cup of hot water.

6 Kali. Phos.

Dip a pad of cotton wool in the brew, squeeze it out and apply to the eyes, then cover the eyes with a folded towel and rest for 10 minutes. It does wonders! You can also sip a hot drink made with six tablets of each of the above salts dissolved in a cup of hot water for a really comforting addition to the treatment.

The ears

Pressure in the ears, and buzzing, roaring or ringing in the ears, often called tinnitus, can be distressing. Here is where Kali. Phos. with Mag. Phos. and Ferrum Phos. come to the rescue, taken as a hot drink together with a gingko biloba tablet. I have found that this 'crisis remedy' calms the panic, eases the pressure and dizziness, and reduces the severity of the noise. To make the drink, dissolve 10 tablets each of Kali. Phos., Mag. Phos. and Ferrum Phos. in a glass of hot water and sip slowly.

The digestive system

When Kali. Phos. is lacking it often shows as a craving for certain foods, even after a big meal. There can be a bitter taste in the mouth and the teeth sometimes chatter.

Kali. Phos. helps with burning indigestion, a feeling of apprehension with butterflies in the stomach, flatulence and colic. Suck two tablets every 30 minutes or so until relief is felt. When there is diarrhoea or dysentery, the combination of Kali. Phos., Calc. Sulph., Mag. Phos. and Nat. Phos. will soon soothe and cleanse. Take two tablets of each salt frequently.

The circulatory system

High blood pressure is often part of the ageing process, but you should never attempt to self-treat this condition. It is imperative to stay on medication prescribed by your doctor. Kali. Phos. and Ferrum Phos. (two tablets of each) will work beautifully together with your medication. If you should feel faint, dizzy or nauseous, take two Kali. Phos. and two Mag. Phos. tablets every 10–30 minutes until you feel easier. This will also help to relieve palpitations, nervous upsets and agitation, and settle an uneven heartbeat. Should the condition persist, see your doctor.

In the case of angina pectoris, suck two tablets of Kali. Phos. and Mag. Phos. frequently daily to help relieve the pain and anxiety, but always stay on medication in consultation with your doctor. When there is fat around the heart, inflamed lungs and pain in the chest, Kali. Phos. and Mag. Phos. are a great comfort. Suck two tablets of each salt frequently, again in conjunction with your prescribed medication.

Gangrene occurs where there is inadequate circulation of blood, usually to an extremity, causing the local tissue to die. Kali. Phos. and Ferrum Phos. tablets are a support; take two of each at least 6–10 times a day. A healing lotion can be made by dissolving 10 tablets each of Kali. Phos. and Ferrum Phos. in a cup of hot water. Spray the lotion onto the affected area frequently and massage it in gently if the skin is unbroken. Keep your doctor informed about your condition.

The respiratory system

Kali. Phos. is very comforting when there is breathlessness, a tight cough, allergic hay fever, nervous or chronic asthma, or a long-term cough. Suck two Kali. Phos. tablets frequently, together with your medications. Ten tablets each of Kali. Phos. and Mag. Phos. dissolved in a glass of hot water will soothe the panic that can rise when gasping for breath. To ease asthmatic wheezing and distress, suck two tablets each of Kali. Phos. and Mag. Phos. every 10 minutes until calm is restored.

The urinary system

In the case of cystitis, take two tablets each of Kali. Phos., Ferrum Phos. and Mag. Phos. frequently, as this formula is soothing and repairing and helps to clear toxins from the bladder.

The skin

Itchy and infected eczema, shingles and rashes all benefit from the wonderfully comforting action of Kali. Phos. and Mag. Phos. Suck two tablets of each every 30 minutes to ease the discomfort. Kali. Phos. is also excellent for a dry, flaky, itchy scalp. To make a soothing skin lotion, dissolve 10 Ferrum Phos., 10 Mag. Phos. and 15 Kali. Phos. tablets in a cup of hot water. Use as a spritz-spray over the area, or dab on as a lotion using a cotton wool pad.

As people age, excessive body odour can become an embarrassing problem, but the remarkable trio of Silica, Nat. Phos. and Kali. Phos. helps alleviate this. In the case of smelly feet, perspiration and bad breath, suck two tablets of each salt frequently, and dissolve 10 of each in a litre of hot water and use as a wash. If you suck the tablets four times a day for 2–4 months, the body odour can be cleared completely.

6 Kali. Phos.

How you feel

We all agree that old age can be challenging. We have to be brave, true to our instincts, and utilise the support of these wonderful little tablets. Remember that Kali. Phos. is one of the tissue salts that eases the fear we may feel about age-related worries such as the fear of illness, incontinence, vision loss, financial problems, insomnia and weakness of the extremities. In addition, there can be remorse, grief, fear of change, disturbing dreams, inability to concentrate, and fear of senility and Alzheimer's disease.

When these fears press upon the once-active senior citizen, suck two tablets each of Kali. Phos., Silica, Ferrum Phos. and Calc. Phos. 2–4 times a day. This will become a ritual you will not want to neglect, especially before switching the light off at night! The salts can also be made into a hot drink and sipped slowly. Crush four tablets each of Kali. Phos., Silica, Ferrum Phos. and Calc. Phos. in a cup of hot water, mix it well and sip slowly.

Some elderly people become reclusive and suspicious, with low energy, mental deterioration and muscle weakness. This indicates lack of Kali. Phos., so reach for the magic formula, which is also a natural tranquiliser. It is so worth exploring these gentle ways of rebuilding. A homeopathic doctor may add valerian, anacardium and alumina to restore body and mind to a more positive space with Kali. Phos. Also check for the presence of danger foods (such as sugar and processed foods) and include abundant fresh fruit and vegetables in the diet.

Other ailments

Chronic fatigue can happen easily, especially in times of stress. Reach for Kali. Phos., Calc. Phos. and Ferrum Phos. when there is nervous exhaustion, forgetfulness, inattentiveness and heavy thoughts and mood. Two tablets of each taken frequently will greatly relieve these symptoms.

Kali. Phos. is hugely important after a stroke. There may be confusion, panic, fear, sensitivity to noise, hysteria, vertigo, palpitations and weak eyesight. Two Kali. Phos. tablets taken every 20–30 minutes, or even every 10 minutes, will soothe things considerably and act as a tonic. Make a hot drink by dissolving 10 tablets each of Kali. Phos., Mag. Phos. and Ferrum Phos. in a cup of hot water and sip slowly, as this will calm the distress and lift the exhaustion.

A lot of work has been done to see whether Kali. Phos. may help to restore and stabilise the nerve sheaths in the early stages of multiple sclerosis. The dosage here would be two tablets up to 10 times a day, which will also help with sleeplessness.

Some European doctors believe that Kali. Phos. has a preventive and protective action in terms of cancer, as in their view certain cancers are caused by a potassium imbalance. These doctors recommend herbs and foods rich in Kali. Phos. and Kali. Mur. in the daily diet, and a drastic reduction in table salt.

Secondary and complementary tissue salts

Kali. Phos. works well with Mag. Phos. as an analgesic, anti-inflammatory and sedative. Kali. Phos. with Calc. Phos. taken together, two tablets of each at a time, helps to 'tone' the skin, the blood and the muscles. Calc. Phos. helps where there is lack of elasticity in the structure of the tissues, and Kali. Phos. is essential where there is no tone, possibly because the nerve supply to the tissues may be weak, partially lacking or even absent.

Another helpful partner to Kali. Phos. is Ferrum. Phos., and these two strong tissue salts make an excellent combination for improving circulation.

Kali. Phos. salad

SERVES 4

This quick, easy salad is delicious and calming, and should be eaten often.

1 cup finely shredded butter lettuce
1 cup finely shredded kale
1 cup finely shredded Swiss chard spinach
1 cup finely shredded cabbage, specially the outer leaves
Lemon juice
Fresh thyme
Chives, chopped
Radishes, chopped
Olives, stoned and pitted
Ginger root, grated
Dates, chopped

Mix the butter letttuce, kale, Swiss chard, spinach and cabbage together and dress with lemon juice, thyme and chives, and add sliced radishes. Top the salad with olives, ginger root and even a few dates. This dish can be enjoyed fresh as a salad or lightly stir-fried.

Herbs that contain Kali. Phos.

Chives (*Allium schoenoprasum*) and **garlic** (*Allium sativum*): These two are excellent expectorants. They are rich in Kali. Phos. and also contain anticoagulant and antibiotic substances. Both reduce high cholesterol, boost the immune system and reduce blood-sugar levels, and should be included in the daily diet. Giant chives and Welsh spring onions have the same properties. All are easy to grow and can be chopped fresh into soups, stews, salads and home-baked breads.

Ginger (*Zingiber officinale*): The root of this delicious herb should be used fresh and finely grated. A teaspoonful in a cup of boiling water with a slice of lemon and a little honey is excellent to lower high blood pressure and to treat coughs, colds, asthma and a tight chest. Ginger is a wonderful anti-inflammatory, a stimulant to the circulatory system, and it eases the digestive system and nausea.

Horseradish (*Armoracia rusticana*): This herb contains Kali. Phos. in both the root and leaves, and it works as a stimulant on the cardiovascular and digestive systems. Finely grated root is a superb antibacterial, with tonic properties and strong anticancer protective qualities. Horseradish opens the sinuses, works against flu, coughs, colds and blocked sinuses, and it has the marvellous ability to stimulate the endorphins, making you feel good all over! It is very worth growing your own.

Mustard (*Brassica alba*): Grow your own mustard and eat the tasty leaves in your daily salad. Mustard is good for the digestion, for the circulation and as a general tonic, and the leaves, flowers and seeds may be eaten. Mix the seeds with honey to make a healthy spread that acts as a digestive stimulant and a vitamin- and mineral-rich warming tonic.

Red clover (*Trifolium pratense*): I cannot stress enough how valuable red clover is as an important anticancer herb. Rich in Kali. Phos. and Mag. Phos., it is a delicious salad ingredient, full of antispasmodic, anti-inflammatory and anti-arthritic properties. It soothes respiratory ailments, eases arthritis, rheumatic pains, spasms, aching muscles and stiff joints, and relieves eczema and psoriasis. Grow red clover abundantly for your daily salad – the more you cut it, the more it grows! I call it a perennial jewel, and the beautiful pink flowers are edible too and are packed with goodness!

St. John's Wort (*Hypericum perforatum*): Rich in phosphorus and potassium, St. John's Wort is a wonderful anti-inflammatory, a gentle sedative and a natural positivity builder that eases aches and pains, and restores the anxious and overwrought nervous system. It is worth growing so that you can make your own tea.

Thyme (*Thymus vulgaris*): A natural antibiotic like the onion family, thyme also has antibacterial, antiseptic and antiviral properties. I enjoy fresh thyme so much that I sprinkle it onto salads, scrambled eggs, pastas, fritters, soups and stews daily, and grow it close to the kitchen door for easy picking. Thyme is excellent for treating bronchitis, as it helps to increase blood flow to the stressed area. It also eases coughing and a tight chest, heals skin ailments, clears infections and is a trusted friend in every dish!

Kali. Phos. stir-fry

SERVES 4

Make this easy supper dish often – you will find that you'll never grow tired of it!

1 cup chopped onions and their green tops
½ cup olive oil
1 cup broccoli florets
2 cups thinly shredded kale leaves
2 cups thinly sliced spinach leaves
6 radishes, thinly sliced – stems and leaved included
2 large potatoes, peeled and diced and cooked in boiling water
    until tender
1 or 2 cloves garlic, finely chopped
Juice of 1 lemon
Himalayan salt and ground black pepper to taste

Fry the onions in olive oil in a large frying pan until just starting to brown, then add all the other ingredients except the lemon juice and seasoning and stir-fry until tender, turning all the time. Then add the lemon juice and seasoning. Serve with slices of steamed fish or grilled chicken.

Foods rich in Kali. Phos.

The following foods are rich in Kali. Phos.: leafy green vegetables (lettuce, spinach, amaranth, beetroot tops, radish root and leaves, green mustard leaves, mustard spinach), green beans, lentils, olives, oats, onions, garlic, cauliflower, broccoli, potatoes, tomatoes, guavas, lemons, cherries, apples, dates, cabbage (outer leaves particularly), kale and walnuts. Growing your own 'Kali. Phos garden' like I do will give you endless pleasure.

Kali. Phos.-rich beetroot bake

SERVES 4

Beetroot, beetroot leaves and organically grown sweet potato are rich in Kali. Phos. Prepare this dish when you have fresh young beetroot.

8 beetroots
6–8 sweet potatoes
4 tablespoons olive oil
1 or 2 tablespoons balsamic vinegar
1½ teaspoons wholegrain mustard
1 teaspoon cornflour
Butter

Preheat the oven to 200°C. Scrub the beetroots and peel with a potato peeler if the skin is too thick – although it's best to leave the skin on. Cut the root and leaves off and slice the beetrot into wedges. Scrub the sweet potatoes and slice into rings. Simmer in boiling water for 10–15 minutes or until soft, then drain. Drizzle olive oil and balsamic vinegar on the beetroot wedges and roast in a pan in the oven for 20–30 minutes until soft and tender. Mash the sweet potatoes with the wholegrain mustard to a fine texture. Remove the roasted beetroot from the roasting pan and place into a baking dish. Add 3 tablespoons of hot water to deglaze the roasting pan, add the cornflour and stir until the sauce thickens. Pour this over the beetroot in the baking dish. Cover the beetroot with the sweet potato mash and dot with a touch of butter. Bake until the sweet potato becomes lightly golden and crunchy. Serve hot with a salad.

This tasty vegetarian dish is rich in nutrients and delicious enough to serve as a party dish.

7 _Kali. Sulph._

Potassium Sulphate • Sulphate of Potash • _Kalium Sulphuricum_

Kali. Sulph.'s main function is as a distributor of oxygen, primarily to the lungs and skin. It helps to keep all the membranes of the body healthy and strengthens the delicate membranes where the exchange of oxygen and carbon dioxide occurs. It shares the load here with Ferrum Phos.

Kali. Sulph. is needed in the third stage of healing for inflammatory conditions such as bronchitis, whooping cough and pneumonia, when the exudations or catarrhs are slimy, thick, yellow and sticky. It relieves exudations from the nose, larynx, lungs, intestines and skin. Ear, nose and throat blockages, and skin problems including acne and oiliness, all indicate a need for Kali. Sulph. Many common skin conditions such as freckles, old-age liver spots, vitiligo (loss of pigmentation, causing white patches), brown patches, eczema, psoriasis, dandruff and oily hair show the need for this tissue salt.

In my early studies of tissue salts I was surprised by the fact that Kali. Sulph. has an affinity with oil. It is the distributor of oil and when Kali. Sulph. is in short supply in the body, the pores of the skin become clogged, especially on the scalp and face. This can result in eruptions such as eczema and psoriasis and is exasperating. The skin peels off and is dry and nothing seems to ease the condition other than Kali. Sulph. (see p.73 for the cream and lotion recipes).

I also learned early on that lack of Kali. Sulph. is often associated with polyps in the ears, blocked ears and earache, ringworm, changeable moods, aversion to work, and the hot flushes that can plague some menopausal women. Include Kali. Sulph. foods, herbs and teas for almost immediate results; grow these plants for convenience and as a pure organic source, and grow sprouts in the kitchen. It is rewarding and inexpensive. Kali. Sulph. also helps to relieve sugar cravings, which is an added benefit! We need to suck two Kali. Sulph. tablets at least four times a day to realise these benefits.

71

7 Kali. Sulph.

As we age we tend to experience pains in the limbs, headaches and neuralgias. Kali. Sulph. can be a steady relief; suck two tablets frequently (up to 10 times during the day) for those often nameless afflictions.

The skin

Kali. Sulph. helps in the formation of new skin cells and as such it acts as a skin lubricator, keeping the skin smooth and youthful. It is also very supportive in the healing process if there is skin disturbance such as spots, rashes, redness and itchiness of any kind. Suck two Kali. Mur. tablets 5–10 times a day to soothe the skin when there is dry flakiness or a weeping eczema, burning skin, an infected cut or graze, pimples, itchy dry skin or a moist, itchy rash. Use the same tablet dosage when there is dandruff, dry flakes or warts on the scalp, or apply a Kali. Sulph. lotion frequently. This will even help to clear a shaving rash, but needs to be applied often.

Vitiligo (pigment loss), discoloration of the skin and lack of perspiration in response to heat respond well to Kali. Sulph. Diseased conditions of the nails, such as ribbed lines, marks and discoloration can be eased by taking Kali. Sulph. tablets and by rubbing Kali. Sulph. paste into the nail surfaces and around the cuticles. To make the paste, crush 10 Kali. Sulph. tablets in a little hot water and apply at least three times during the day after washing the hands.

Kali. Sulph. also helps with peeling skin (desquamation). It will clear the affected area smoothly, so use a Kali. Sulph. cream liberally, or spread the paste over the area and leave it to dry. Epithelial skin cancers also respond to the cream and paste, as do rashes with exudations and all eruptive diseases. Measles and scarlet fever have been treated successfully with Kali. Sulph., and in the case of ageing skin it is useful for its clearing action.

The ears

When there is thick mucus build-up that seems to block the ears, suck two Kali. Sulph. tablets 6–8 times through the day. This will do much to open blocked ears, especially where there is discharge and chronic catarrh. Polyps in the ears, earache and general ear discomfort are also eased with Kali. Sulph., and a Kali. Sulph. hot drink can be a great comfort. Dissolve 10 Kali. Sulph. tablets in a cup of hot water and sip slowly to ease ear congestion, clear the wax that accompanies the earache and get a good night's sleep.

Kali. Sulph. cream

1½ cups aqueous cream
1 cup fresh green barley grass, chopped
½ cup fresh salad burnet leaves (*Sanguisorba minor*)
½ cup fresh parsley (*Petroselinum crispum*)
3 teaspoons vitamin E oil

In a double boiler, simmer the aqueous cream with the barley grass, salad burnet and parsley for 20 minutes. Mix well and stir frequently. Strain the mixture, working it through a fine sieve. Add the vitamin E oil and mix well. Store in a glass jar with a good screw-top lid.

Kali. Sulph. lotion

1 cup fresh salad burnet leaves (*Sanguisorba minor*)
1 cup fresh parsley (*Petroselinum crispum*)
1 litre water
10 Kali. Sulph. tablets, finely crushed

Simmer the salad burnet, parsley and water in a double boiler for 20 minutes, pressing down well with a heavy spoon. Set the brew aside to cool (keep it covered). Strain, then dissolve the finely crushed Kali. Sulph. tablets in the warm water. Pour into a spritz-spray bottle and use lavishly and often. This will become a much-loved beauty lotion!

The respiratory system

Kali. Sulph. is indicated when there is a thick rattling chest, a phlegmy cough, short breath, craving for fresh cool air, bronchitis, pneumonia, asthma, or a chronic cough with yellow sputum. Suck two tablets frequently. Congestion of the ears, nose and throat, catarrhal deafness, thick postnasal drip and a creamy-yellow coating on the tongue can also be cleared in this way, or dissolve 10–12 Kali. Sulph. tablets in a cup of hot water and sip slowly. Remember that even the eyes can be affected by sinus build-up, coughing and sinus-related migraines, which is where Kali. Sulph. is needed urgently, often alongside medication from your doctor.

The digestive system

Kali. Sulph. comes to the rescue when there is colic, belching, bloating and flatulence with a strong sulphurous odour. Ten tablets dissolved in a cup of hot water and sipped slowly will do much to bring relief. Yellow diarrhoea or thin dark stools, haemorrhoids, and a burning sensation in the rectum and lower bowel are also eased by sipping a Kali. Sulph. drink. To clear sulphurous odour and diarrhoea that is purulent and slimy, try Kali. Sulph. tea: pour 1½ cups of boiling water over ¼ cup melissa and ¼ cup fresh parsley. Let the tea stand for five minutes before straining. Crush 10 Kali. Sulph. tablets and dissolve in the tea. Sip slowly, retaining the tea in the mouth for at least 10 seconds at a time to allow absorption of the beneficial salts and herbs.

The urinary system

Cystitis is a real discomfort for some women, and with age this can become chronic. Here is where Kali. Sulph. is a great friend, taken alongside medication from your doctor. Suck two Kali. Sulph. tablets frequently through the day to clear the discharge. Where there is backache with these symptoms, Kali. Sulph. will ease the tension, pressure and pain.

The circulatory system

Haemorrhoids and throbbing varicose veins can be eased with a Kali. Sulph. wash or cream, and two tablets should be sucked at least eight times through the day. To make the wash, simmer three cups of comfrey leaves in two litres of boiling water (tear the comfrey leaves into small pieces) and stir frequently. Simmer with the lid on for 20 minutes. Cool the lotion to comfortable warmth, strain, and add 10 crushed Kali. Sulph. tablets. Use as a lotion, wash and poultice over the haemorrhoids or varicose veins. Neuralgia of the face also benefits from the above wash. Dip a cloth into the hot brew, wring it out and apply to painful areas on the face or behind the ear. Hold it over the area for as long as is comfortable, and repeat.

Female problems

Kali. Sulph. helps to clear leucorrhoea (white vaginal discharge due to infection). Increase your intake of Kali. Sulph. foods and eliminate sugar, which aggravates the condition, from the diet.

Menopause can be taxing for some women and hot flushes can linger. Kali. Sulph. cools and regulates the frequency of the flushes and helps to smooth and relieve discomfort during menopause and beyond. I have come to rely on it daily to clear up minor congestions and irritations, especially in hot weather where rooms are stuffy. Sip a long glass of cold water with two Kali. Sulph. tablets every 15–20 minutes to ease an overheated system.

Joint pains

In the case of aching joints, non-specific pains and discomfort in the bones, suck two Kali. Sulph. and two Mag. Phos. tablets 8–10 times through the day. This becomes a panacea and needs to be on the bedside table to ensure a painless night. Pain-filled waking in the small hours can get to one as the years pile on, but this bedside formula will soothe, ease and comfort. I find that a small cup of warm milk with a touch of honey and six tablets each of Kali. Sulph. and Mag. Phos. dissolved in it gets me back to sleep again quickly. Sip it slowly and hold it in the mouth for a few seconds before swallowing.

What you feel

When Kali. Sulph. is deficient, emotional symptoms include quick temper, irritability and sensitivity to noise such as loud music and the sound of children playing noisily. There are sometimes disturbing dreams, a need for reassurance and validation, anxiety and sadness. Two Kali. Sulph. tablets taken 3–6 times a day will help to ease these symptoms. Become aware of those anxious feelings and treat them immediately. Interestingly, I find sucking two tablets of Combin 12 (the tablet that combines of all 12 tissue salts) brings immediate relief, and then I continue with Kali. Sulph.

Other ailments

Other physical conditions that benefit from this tissue salt are: fungoid inflammation of the joints; typhoid, typhus and blood poisoning; cancerous spots on the face and backs of the hands; difficulty in swallowing, with a constricted throat; and hot, painful rheumatism. Kali. Sulph. also clears mucus from all parts of the body, especially when combined with Ferrum Phos., Calc. Sulph. and Kali. Sulph.

Lack of potassium has been associated with cancer, and the cancer formula used by some dedicated practitioners is Ferrum Phos., Kali. Mur., Kali. Phos. and Kali. Sulph. (easy to remember as numbers 4, 5, 6 and 7). Two tablets of each should be taken several times daily, even 8–10 times a day in severe cases. There are some remarkable case histories. Cancerous cells on the nose respond well to Kali. Sulph. cream and paste, and under your doctor's supervision this is worth trying.

7 Kali. Sulph.

Thyroid conditions can sometimes indicate a lack of Kali. Sulph., so this is an important tissue salt for the thyroid. High fever, overheating and heat rash all respond to Kali. Sulph., and the lotion used as a spritz-spray is particularly effective in lowering a high temperature (see recipe on p.73). In hot weather, spray it on exposed skin while a fan is on. Homeopathic doctors have found pulsatilla to be an excellent remedy with Kali. Sulph. for the above symptoms.

Wherever there is discharge, from the nose, throat, skin or vagina, Kali. Suph. is the salt to clear it. All three of the Kaliums are extraordinary and often all three can be combined into a profound cleanser.

Secondary and complementary tissue salts

Kali. Mur., Kali. Phos. and Kali. Sulph. work powerfully together – each strengthening and supporting the other, especially clearing old infections of the chest, and, with Ferrum. Phos. clearing any other infections, old mucus can be relatively easily dispelled and cleared.

Ferrum. Phos. is taken for the first stage of an illness. Kali. Mur. then starts the cleansing and healing process in the second stage of the illness (think of bronchitis as a good example). The Kali. Sulph. comes in at the end to clear out all the old mucus and thick, old phlegm that has become sticky and tenacious. This is the third and final stage of the infection.

All three can be taken together even at the onset of a chest infection, as their combined action boosts the healing process that is vital for the elderly patient, who can become weaker if the mucus builds up too fast.

The combination of Kali. Sulph. and Calc. Sulph. – two tablets of each taken three or four times a day – are two of the tissue salts that have been used for treating cancer patients who are in remission. Doctors Carey and Perry found that injections of Kali. Sulph. with Ferrum. Phos. were effective for uterine, intestinal and vaginal cancer. The oral dosage is two tablets each of Ferrum Phos. and Kali. Sulph. taken 6–8 times a day. Always discuss your treatment with your doctor and follow their advice.

Herbs that contain Kali. Sulph.

Linseed/Flax (*Linum usitatissimum*): We underestimate the power of the humble linseed. It is rich in Kali. Sulph. as well as vitamins A, B, C and E, and it has antiseptic, antirheumatic, laxative and diuretic properties, and breaks down mucus build-up. Two or three teaspoons of linseed with breakfast oats will soothe the digestive tract, act as a natural laxative and dissolve mucus in the alimentary canal. It can also be grown as a sprout and mixed with apple and papaya for breakfast when there is constipation. Linseed becomes jelly-like when wet and this acts as a gentle laxative.

Melissa or lemon balm (*Melissa officinalis*): This wonderful herb lessens tension, anxiety, fear and shakiness, and eases and tones the digestive system. It relaxes the peripheral blood vessels, and has antiviral, antibacterial and antispasmodic properties. Melissa makes one of the most healing digestive teas I know: pour a cup of boiling water over ¼ cup fresh sprigs, stir well, let the tea stand for five minutes, stir again, strain and sip slowly.

Mustard (*Brassica nigra*): Mustard has strong cleansing, rejuvenating qualities and makes a quick and easy-to-grow sprout, micro-green and plant in the garden. It is rich in vitamins, minerals and enzymes, and should be eaten in salads and stir-fries as a boost to the circulation, a detoxifier, a kidney and bladder tonic, and to clear up old coughs, chesty mucus and slow-healing wounds.

Parsley (*Petroselinum crispum*): This is one of the most amazing herbs, one we should be eating daily as we grow older! It is a cleanser, detoxifier and diuretic, and flushes the system, as it is rich in Kali. Sulph. The liver, lungs, kidneys, bladder and circulatory system all benefit from eating fresh parsley daily, and parsley tea is a boon for old coughs, mucus and chesty wheezing with feelings of suffocation. Eat it finely chopped on savoury dishes, from scrambled eggs to soups and stews. It is worth growing both moss-curled parsley and the flat-leaf Italian parsley all year round near the kitchen door for quick picking.

Salad burnet (*Sanguisorba officinalis*): Rich in Kali. Sulph., salad burnet is an almost forgotten herb that we need to grow for its cleansing diuretic action and its ability to clear toxins from the liver in particular. It also has antibacterial, antiseptic and diuretic properties, and it is rich in minerals, particularly potassium, which we need more of as we age. Its mild, easily digested leaves taste of cucumber and are delicious in salads and stir-fries.

Watercress (*Nasturtium officinale*): Rich in iron, potassium, phosphorus and vitamins A, B_1, B_2, C and E, this easy-to-grow winter herb requires just a moist position in partial shade and will produce an abundant spring crop. It clears old mucus and chesty build-up and cleanses superbly. A salad made with watercress sprigs and young mustard leaves dressed with lemon juice will build up a depleted system quickly after winter coughs and colds.

Home-made muesli

Rich in many vitamins, minerals and Kali. Sulph., this is a sustaining and energising breakfast for every day.

4 cups large flake oats (non-instant)
2 cups husked sunflower seeds
2 cups sundried mixed cranberries, sultanas and blueberries
2 cups chopped apple rings (dried in a dryer)
½ cup chopped almonds, walnuts, pecan nuts

Mix everything together and store in a glass jar with a good screw-top lid in the refrigerator. Shake it up every now and then. Pour out enough for breakfast each morning and eat with a little warmed plain Bulgarian yoghurt and fresh fruit (such as grated apple, fresh mango slices, papaya or mashed banana).

Foods rich in Kali. Sulph.

Plain Greek or Bulgarian yoghurt is rich in vitamins, minerals and calcium, and in small amounts will help to relieve lactose intolerance, improve the digestion and support healthy gut bacteria. Just a little for breakfast with oats and goji berries will spark up the day!

Barley is a wonder food, rich in Kali. Sulph. The grains can be sprouted and the young barley grass juiced. It is packed with vitality, vitamins and minerals. To make health-giving barley water, simmer a cup of pearl barley in two litres of water for about 20 minutes. Use a stainless steel pot. Keep topping up the water, as it boils away quite quickly. Strain and eat the barley like rice, and keep the liquid chilled and covered in the fridge. Pour a glass or two daily and serve cold with slices of lemon and lemon juice and fresh stevia leaves for sweetness. It will lower cholesterol and cleanse the system. Let this become a daily drink.

Freshly grated carrots are rich in Kali. Sulph. and make a lovely salad. Look for organically grown ones or grow your own. Lettuce, endives, chicory, lemons, almonds and rye (grow it like barley grass and also sprout it) are also rich in this tissue salt, as are lentils, spinach, peas and pea flowers and leaves, pecan nuts, walnuts, hazelnuts and cottage cheese.

Learn to bake your own wholemeal pan bread and add linseeds, chopped walnuts or almonds to it. My daughter Sandy has mastered this delicious Kali. Sulph.-rich bread and she serves it in her restaurant at the Herbal Centre. It is quick, easy and rewarding!

Sandy's pan bread

2 cups wholemeal brown bread flour (we use Eureka flours, which
    are organically grown and processed)
½ cup plain yoghurt mixed into 1 cup warm water
2 teaspoons baking powder
½ teaspoon salt
2 tablespoons linseeds
1 cup mustard sprouts

Mix all the ingredients together. Heat a non-Teflon pan to medium heat; we use a 'green' pan with a ceramic coating. Add about a tablespoon of olive oil and coat the pan evenly. Tip the bread mixture into the pan and spread with a spatula. Shake the pan frequently to prevent burning and do not leave it unattended. When the mixture starts to bubble, place a well-oiled flat plate over the pan and flip it over. Re-oil the pan and slide the bread back into the pan so that the uncooked side is facing down.

Keep shaking the pan to disperse the heat and add a little more olive oil if needed. When the bread sounds hollow when tapped, it is done. It is easy, quick, delicious and healthy as there are no chemicals in it. Serve hot with butter and salads; I grow summer tomatoes and cucumbers to eat with it. Practice makes perfect but it is worth it as this bread is a jewel!

8 Mag. Phos.

Magnesium Phosphate • Phosphate of Magnesia • Magnesia Phosphorica

Mag. Phos. is a highly effective spasm reliever and cramp treatment. Many athletes have found it to be wonderfully soothing, and I use Mag. Phos. abundantly in the creams I make for physiotherapists.

Nerves and muscles are composed of many strands of fibres; surprisingly, they are of many different shades or colours. The white fibres within the nerves and muscles have an affinity for Mag. P hos., and absorb it by molecular action. When there is a deficiency in this cell salt, this is indicated by spasm or cramp.

Let us consider colic or stomachache. When there is a Mag. Phos. deficiency the muscular walls of the stomach contract and 'cramp', reducing the cavity of the stomach. Gas forms to prevent a collapse of the stomach and thus serves as a 'counterforce'. Suck two Mag. Phos. tablets every 3–5 minutes to relieve the pain; should this not provide immediate relief, suck two Calc. Phos. tablets to release the spasm and ease the discomfort.

I have found that a night-time headache can be avoided by sucking two Mag. Phos. tablets in the late afternoon and two before bedtime. I also increase my daily water consumption, as this goes well with extra Mag. Phos., and take omega-3 and -6 oil capsules as well. Other headache sufferers have confirmed that this has helped them too. The omega oils help to ease pain, and for the chronic aches and pains of ageing, this is something we need to consider.

Involuntary twitches, jerks, spasms and limb movements, once known as 'St Vitus dance', can be eased, if not cured, with dedicated use of Mag. Phos. It is an exceptional remedy for spasmodic illnesses, including some heart ailments, as well as writer's cramp, shaking hands, a shaky jaw and chattering teeth at times of distress and shock.

It is also a good analgesic, and is also perfect for a range of conditions, from persistent hiccups to heart palpitations. There is seemingly no end to its uses!

The head

When there are headaches, often with sharp shooting or throbbing pain, visual disturbance, a feeling of being cross-eyed, or neuralgia of the face, Ferrum Phos. and Mag. Phos. work exceptionally well together. Two tablets of each sucked frequently bring relief without leaving one feeling listless and drowsy, which can happen with heavy medication. Neuralgia of the face, neck or scalp and trembling of the head can be eased by taking two Mag. Phos. tablets every 15 minutes until the condition eases.

In the case of lockjaw, anti-tetanus injections are vital and should be renewed with your doctor every few years. Take Mag. Phos. frequently together with your doctor's medication, as it will help to clear the infection. Spasmodic stammering, twitches and spasms of the lips, and spontaneous face pulling all need Mag. Phos. To make a hot drink, dissolve 10 tablets each of Mag. Phos. and Kali. Phos. in a cup of hot (boiled) water and hold in the mouth for a few seconds before swallowing.

The eyes

In the case of blurred vision, a spontaneous tic or occipital neuralgia, suck two Mag. Phos. tablets as needed every 5–20 minutes. A hot Mag. Phos. compress can also be applied to the temples, eyes and head, and is wonderfully soothing. To make it, dissolve 10 Mag. Phos. tablets in a cup of hot water. Boil the water first, then cool to a comfortable warmth. Add 10 Ferrum Phos. tablets if the eyes are itchy, sore, red or feeling scratchy. Dip cotton wool pads in the hot mixture, squeeze them out and wipe over the closed eyes, or use as a poultice, replacing with new pads frequently. Dull eyes, blurred sight, drooping eyelids and constricted pupils do well with Mag. Phos. and Kali. Phos. together. Take two tablets of each every 20 minutes.

The ears

For earache caused by middle ear inflammation (otitis media), take two Mag. Phos. tablets every 15 minutes until you can get to your doctor. Do not try to treat earache on your own. Mag. Phos. is also very helpful taken every 10–15 minutes when hearing is dull and there is aching all around the ears, as well as ringing in the ears that is spasmodic and not caused by an infection. I often use Mag. Phos. when I cannot distinguish sounds (too much noise often confuses) or when there is hearing impairment. Here is where Mag. Phos. is soothing and needs to be taken regularly. It is one of the most important remedies for hearing impairment caused by nervous tension.

8 Mag. Phos.

The nose

Loss of sense of smell that is not connected to a cold suggests a Mag. Phos. deficiency. Suck two Mag. Phos. tablets at least five times through the day, and persist with the treatment. This is often a symptom that bewilders ageing women far more than men. It responds well to Mag. Phos.

The throat

Where there is convulsive coughing, Mag. Phos. is a panacea. Spasmodic breathlessness, choking when attempting to swallow, constricted feeling in the throat, and a tight cough when talking are indicative of Mag. Phos. deficiency. A sudden shrill voice when speaking or singing (throat spasm) benefits from Kali. Phos. with Mag. Phos.; six tablets of each dissolved in half a cup of hot water and sipped slowly will ease the windpipe beautifully. Also gargle a little and then swallow.

Oral and facial health

Teeth that are sensitive to cold or to touch indicate a lack of Mag. Phos. When there is neuralgia of the face, shooting pains, spasmodic pain and even rheumatic pain relieved by warmth, Mag. Phos. is the treatment. However, if a cold (rather than hot) compress relieves the pain, then Ferrum Phos. is indicated rather than Mag. Phos. as Ferrum Phos. relieves inflammatory conditions of the nerves and adjacent tissues.

The digestive system

Two Mag. Phos. tablets sucked every 10 minutes will ease heartburn, colic, indigestion, flatulence and bloating, and will also help to quell hunger pangs. Lack of magnesium is often connected with severe diarrhoea, bowel cramps, stomach cramps, chronic pain around the liver (check with your doctor as this could be a chronic liver disease possibly caused by rich food and alcoholism), irritable bowel syndrome, spastic colon, Crohn's disease and bloated colic.

When there are hiccups, vomiting with griping pains, or if the pain is spasmodic with belching, sip a hot Mag. Phos. and Ferrum Phos. drink (10 tablets of each dissolved in a cup of hot boiled water), holding the mixture in the mouth for five seconds before swallowing. It will immediately soothe and release the tension and pain.

In the case of dysentery, when there are frequent watery stools with mucus and blood in them, you must consult a doctor. Ten tablets each of Kali. Mur. and Mag. Phos. should be dissolved into a cup of hot (boiled) water and sipped slowly until you can get to the doctor, but do not delay, and be sure to drink lots of water. In all cases of diarrhoea, bowel spasms and watery stools, normal absorption needs to be restored. Also ask your doctor about probiotics.

Mag. Phos. helps to keep the blood alkaline, and the digestive process is protected and kept in normal functioning mode, restoring the patient gently, effectively and thoroughly. Nat. Phos. can be added as an antacid, and I have found the combination of Mag. Phos. and Nat. Phos. so valuable that I include them daily in my diet.

Sugar craving

Sugar craving can colour the day; frequently a whole slab of chocolate is not enough to satisfy it! The craving often arises after a meal. This 'sweet-tooth syndrome' clearly indicates a Mag. Phos. deficiency. Suck two tablets every time you need a sugar fix and persist, as it may take a few days to clear. Mag. Phos. will also ease the craving for sweet carbonated cooldrinks, especially colas. Also, change to fresh or dried stevia leaves, which are 300 times sweeter than sugar, but much healthier.

The urinary system

Retention of urine is uncomfortable, often painful and frustrating. Alternate Mag. Phos. and Ferrum Phos. to ease the spasms and restore good balance. When there is strain while urinating or when kidney stones are beginning to develop, dissolve six tablets each of Kali. Phos., Mag. Phos. and Ferrum Phos. in a cup of hot (boiled) water and sip frequently. Add 10 Nat. Sulph. tablets to the formula when kidney stones are being passed. The secret is to sip the drink frequently (keep the mixture in a Thermos flask as the warmth soothes, sip a little at a time, and get to your doctor).

Include Mag. Phos. daily if there is a stricture in the urethra, a swollen prostate gland or difficulty passing urine. Remember the golden rule: you can take tissue salts frequently and you cannot overdose!

Female problems

Painful periods and passing of large clots can be eased with Mag. Phos., Kali. Phos. and Ferrum Phos. Dissolve six tablets of each in ½–1 cup of hot water and sip slowly 3–5 times a day to ease excessive bleeding and pain. When the 'change of life' is under way and discomfort occurs, add eight Calc. Fluor. tablets to the formula to ease the discomfort.

How you feel

Mag. Phos. helps enormously with mood swings, agitation, angry outbursts, touchiness, blaming others, irregular heartbeat and poor sleep patterns. Suck two Mag. Phos. tablets every 10 minutes until you feel calm.

Mag. Phos. also helps quickly when there is crying, stammering, and embarrassing situations with shock and fear. Suck two tablets every five minutes for at least 20–30 minutes. In general, when there is a sense of not coping or the desolation of ageing, keep a bottle of Mag. Phos. near at hand.

Mag. Phos. is equally important for those who sit motionless, lost in thought, and those who pace restlessly, and if it is taken with Kali. Phos. it will help to lift the spirits and restore equilibrium.

Emotional rescue

A really helpful formula is six tablets each of Mag. Phos., Kali. Phos., Ferrum Phos. and Nat. Phos. dissolved in a cup of hot water. Sip slowly and take deep breaths between sips. This marvellously positive combination will restore balance to those who feel ageing is getting the better of them. I often say: 'Write it in your heart' so you do not forget it, as it will calm, collect and concentrate. It is safe for the young and the very elderly – so this formula is a little lifesaver!

Other ailments

In the case of chest pains, call a doctor immediately! Suck two Mag. Phos. tablets every 5–10 minutes until you can get to a doctor as this will help to ease the intensity of the pain. When there is exhaustion, extreme fatigue and a quivery shaky feeling, suck two Mag. Phos. tablets every 10 minutes, and put your feet up until you feel steady.

This is the tissue salt that soothes all cramps within two minutes. I have it on my bedside table, and take it when travelling, playing a musical instrument and when writing for long hours, as this can make me 'crampy' from the neck and shoulders down to the feet! Dissolve 10 Mag. Phos. tablets in half a cup of hot water and sip it frequently. It is a great comfort and relief.

Mag. Phos. eases late-onset diabetic ailments, spasmodic coughing, breathlessness, convulsions, sciatic nerve pains down the leg, and lower back pain. It also helps with alcohol addiction. To my mind, Mag. Phos. is a type of Rescue Remedy, and I have formulated a unique de-stressing and coping tablet, which I call 'crisis remedy', that I post countrywide. This will ease restless sleep, Parkinson's tremors, night terrors, cold sweats, muscle twitching and limb jerking, nausea, vomiting, intense worry, and even Tourette's syndrome.

Where there is sunburn, mosquito bites, itching and swelling, Mag. Phos. comes to the rescue. Make a lotion by dissolving 10 crushed Mag. Phos. tablets in a cup of boiling water, cooled to a comfortable temperature. Either dab the lotion on using pads of cotton wool, or spritz-spray it onto the area. Also, suck two Mag. Phos. tablets frequently. This will calm, soothe and restore you to a better space. Mag. Phos. is also important in treating the pains of arthritis and rheumatism, particularly if the pains are sharp and stabbing – do not forget it for ageing horses and dogs too!

For dizzy spells, lack of balance, and if there has been a fall or concussion, suck two Mag. Phos. tablets every 10 minutes or dissolve 10 in a cup of hot water. When there is an inability to concentrate and forgetfulness, Mag. Phos. helps quickly. Suck two tablets before attending an important function, and even during it, as it helps one to remember names and important points!

Secondary and complementary tissue salts

Mag. Phos. combines well with Kali. Phos. to produce a 'feel-good' state. Suck two tablets of each every five minutes to ease stress, nervous exhaustion, pain and muscular spasm. When your legs do not seem to hold you up, add Calc. Phos. to make an excellent little formula for both pain and anxiety reduction!

Herbs than contain Mag. Phos.

Chamomile (*Chamomilla recutita*): This is a de-stressing herb. Grow it in winter for use throughout the year as a calming tea. To make a tea, pour a cup of boiling water over ¼ cup fresh or dried flowers; let it stand for five minutes, stir well, strain and sip slowly. Chamomile is also wonderful in a hot bath to unwind and release tension after a stressful day. Pour a litre of boiling water over a cup of fresh or dried flowers, let it stand for 20 minutes, then strain and add the water to your bath.

Dandelion (*Taraxacum officinale*): A few fresh leaves a day added to the daily salad works wonders, building bones, cleansing the liver, aiding the digestion, and acting as an antirheumatic. Use young leaves, as older leaves develop a more bitter taste. Dandelion is also rich in vitamins A, B, C and D, and its detoxifying action clears painful spasms.

Dill (*Anthemum graveolens*): Rich in Mag. Phos., dill makes an excellent tea. To make the tea, pour a cup of boiling water over one teaspoon of dill seeds or ¼ cup fresh dill leaves and flowers, and stir well. Let the tea stand for five minutes, then strain. Dry dill seeds for use in the winter months.

Melissa/lemon balm/lemon mint (*Melissa officinalis*): This is most definitely a herb worth growing for all stages of our lives, especially when we are anxious, shaky and not coping! To make a healing tea, pour a cup of boiling water over ¼ cup sprigs; let it stand for five minutes, stir well, strain and sip slowly.

Mints: The *Mentha* varieties are rich in Mag. Phos., especially peppermint. All have antispasmodic and analgesic qualities. To make a tea, pour a cup of boiling water over ¼ cup sprigs; let it stand for five minutes, stir well, strain and sip slowly.

Nettle (*Urtica dioica*): Nettle is rich in magnesium and can be made into a tea by pouring a cup of boiling water over ¼ cup of fresh herb; let the tea stand for five minutes, strain and sip slowly.

Sage (*Salvia officinalis*): Sage is rich in Mag. Phos. and a host of minerals and vitamins. It makes a great treatment for sore throats and coughs; chop it finely and mix it with equal quantities of honey and lemon juice. Sage also relaxes peripheral blood vessels, reduces blood sugar levels, lowers high temperatures and clears heat from the body. It is also a natural antiseptic.

Foods rich in Mag. Phos.

The following whole foods are rich in Mag. Phos.: green leafy vegetables and lettuces, garden peas, apples, plums, oranges, grapefruit, lemons, bananas, figs (fresh and dried), lentils, dried beans, seeds, sprouts, almonds and walnuts.

Tasty sprouts include mung beans, fenugreek, mustard, buckwheat, sesame seed, sunflower seeds and chickpeas. Grow these for salads, blend them with apple juice, figs and bananas. Eat almonds and walnuts as snacks. The Mag. Phos.-rich grains such as wheatgrass, barley grass, millet, dill and oats can all be sprouted, and oat grass is excellent for osteoporosis and joint pains. Inclusion of these foods means extra energy, vitality and ease of movement for the senior citizen!

Oat grass tea

This beverage is delicious and Is wonderful for building bones and for treating osteoporosis.

½ cup rip dry oat grass pieces (about 2cm long)
1 cup boiling water

Pour the boiling water over the oat grass pieces. Let it stand for five minutes, stirring and pressing the oat grass pieces thoroughly. Strain and sip it slowly.
   This tea can be used as a delicious cool-drink base. Add a litre of chilled fresh apple juice to a litre of cooled oat grass tea and serve it with ice.

Oat straw and mint tea

4 cups chopped oats straw (it needs to be dried and the colour of parchment)
2 litres boiling water
6 slices fresh ginger
5 thumb-length sprigs fresh spearmint/peppermint

Simmer the oats straw in the boiled water for 10 minutes. Add the ginger and mint and stir in thoroughly. Cover and set it aside to cool. Strain and sweeten if liked with a touch of honey. Sip slowly, holding the liquid in the mouth briefly before swallowing. This tea combines fabulously with the Mag. Phos. snack food, giving abundant energy.

Mag. Phos. snack food

This quick, energising snack is excellent when you need a boost. It is best to dry your own fruit in a dryer, if possible.

3 cups apple rings
3 cups chopped dried figs
2 cups dried mulberries, blackberries, raspberries, cranberries
2 cups dried naartjie segments (dried without the skin of the segment)
2 cups dried mango slices
1 cup chopped dried ginger slices (steep in stevia syrup before drying)
2 cups almonds
3 cups pecan nuts

Mix all the fruit and nuts in an airtight container and grab a handful when you need a healthy snack. I have also dried thin slices of sweet plum and added this to vary it from time to time. Buying a dryer with tiers of drying trays has been one of my best investments.

9 Nat. Mur.

Sodium Chloride (salt) • Chloride of Soda • *Natrum Muriaticum*

Nat. Mur. regulates the moisture content in every cell in the body and distributes water throughout the system. Lack of this vital salt shows as excessive dryness or excessive moisture, such as swelling in the feet and lower legs. However, do not think that an imbalance can be restored merely by adding extra table salt to food. This will only exacerbate the problem, as the cells cannot utilise the salt unless the particles are available in the attenuated homeopathic form of the actual Nat. Mur. tissue salt. People on a salt-free diet can therefore take Nat. Mur. in complete safety.

If you consider that two-thirds of the body is made up of water, you can understand the vital role that Nat. Mur. plays in maintaining health. That is why eating foods rich in Nat. Mur. is so important, and even essential for us as we age. Without Nat. Mur., the body's normal growth and function is compromised and ailments can become evident, often daily. Consider the many common conditions caused by Nat. Mur. deficiency (described below) and keep that precious little bottle of tablets near at hand!

The skin

I find Nat. Mur. to be exceptional on the skin, and over the years have kept extensive records of its role in the healing of chronic and often debilitating skin conditions. The skin cream recipe on p.90 will help to relieve the cracks, flakes, itches and weeping skin of psoriasis, which is considered a complex and difficult condition to manage.

The cream will also help to heal sunburn, itchy crusty hives, nail fungus, weeping eczema, dry facial skin, blisters, rashes, fine white scales on the skin, and raised red insect bites such as swollen mosquito bites. For all these skin ailments take Nat. Mur. tablets frequently, and use it in the skin cream and as a lotion (10 tablets dissolved in a cup of boiled water).

Nat. Mur. skin cream

2 cups good aqueous cream
½ cup chopped comfrey (*Symphytum officinale*) leaves
½ cup chopped violet (*Viola odorata*) leaves and flowers if in
   bloom
½ cup calendula (*Calendula officinalis*) petals
½ cup chopped buckwheat (*Fagopyrum esculentum*) leaves
   and flowers
1 tablespoon grapeseed oil
3 teaspoons vitamin E oil
1 tablespoon sesame oil
1 tablespoon almond oil
20 Nat. Mur., 10 Ferrum Phos. and 10 Kali. Phos. tablets, crushed

Simmer the aqueous cream, comfrey, violet, calendula and buckwheat
in a double boiler. Use a heavy spoon to press the herbs down well
against the sides of the pot to extract all the juice. Simmer the mixture
for 20 minutes. Allow it to cool, and strain out the herbs (tie them in a
piece of cheese cloth and toss it into the bath or use the little bundle
with soap as a scrub over aching feet and legs). Add the grapeseed,
vitamin E, sesame and almond oils and mix in well. Finally, add the
crushed tissue salts and stir thoroughly. Spoon the cream into screw-top
glass jars, label and store in the fridge. This is one of the most effective
creams I make.

Oily skin and acne respond well to Nat. Mur. and this tissue salt is a
wonderfully soothing treatment for incessant itching. When there is
shingles with a burning feeling, dissolve 10 tablets each of Nat. Mur. and
Mag. Phos. in a cup of hot water and sip it slowly, or let the lotion cool and
use it as a spritz-spray over the area. Alternate this lotion with the fresh
juice of bulbinella (*Bulbine frutescens*), which can be squeezed directly onto
the skin. This is one of the few ways to ease the pain and burning sensation
of shingles.

   A particularly comforting formula is two tablets each of Nat. Mur., Kali.
Mur. and Kali. Phos. taken 3–6 times a day, together with Calc. Phos. and
Ferrum Phos. three times a day. Take this formula with chamomile and
garden violet tea, which is especially soothing for older people. The tea can

also be cooled and used as a spray on the skin. The above regimen needs to be kept up on a daily basis for two weeks to clear the last stages of shingles.

The head

Headaches requiring Nat. Mur. typically begin after a night of poor sleep and peak around noon. At the first hint of a headache, suck two tablets each of Nat. Mur. and Mag. Phos. every 10 minutes; if you do this for about an hour the headache will usually dissipate. Make sure that your body is well hydrated and drink an ample amount of water.

The eyes and nose

In the case of dry itchy eyes, cataracts, 'watery' eyes, itchy eyelids, bags under the eyes, and general puffiness around the eyes, suck two Nat. Mur. tablets every 15 minutes to ease the condition. A soothing lotion can be made by dissolving 10 Nat. Mur. tablets in half a cup of hot water. Dip cotton wool pads in the lotion, squeeze them out gently and use as a wipe or pad over the eyes while you relax for a few minutes. Keep using fresh pads and discarding the used ones. This really brings comfort to the eyes.

Nat. Mur. is one of the flu formula tissue salts (numbers 1, 4, 5, 9 and 11), so remember it at the beginning of a cold or flu when there is copious watery nasal catarrh. At the other extreme, when there is a dry nose, scratchy dry eyes, double vision with a headache, and the eyes feel weak, suck two Nat. Mur. tablets every 10 minutes. When windy weather conditions cause the eyes to smart, wipe the eyes with the Nat. Mur. lotion (above) and suck two Nat. Mur. tablets to ease the discomfort quickly.

Oral health

When there are clear map marks on the tongue (known as geographic tongue), and bleeding gums or mouth ulcers with irritability, Nat. Mur. taken with Calc. Fluor. is often a quick-fix remedy. This combination also works well for a dry mouth, dribbling, cracked corners of the mouth, and even vertical lines on dry lips. For these conditions, I find a Nat. Mur. hot drink very soothing, taken at night, on rising, and once or twice through the day. Crush and dissolve 10 Nat. Mur. tablets in half a cup of hot water and take sips, holding the hot 'tea' in the mouth for as long as is comfortable before swallowing.

I also use this 'tea' for fever blisters (*Herpes simplex* virus), alternating with a tea of elderflowers and black peppermint (see *My 100 Favourite Herbs* for further information). To make the latter, pour a cup of boiling water over ¼ cup each of fresh elderflowers and peppermint (*Mentha piperita nigra* – it needs to be this particular mint) and let it draw for five minutes. I also dissolve 10 Nat. Mur. tablets in the tea and sip it slowly. It is worth growing the elder tree and black peppermint to help clear this condition. Do not forget this, for as we age we want to be free of the little niggles that Nat. Mur. herbs and tablets clear so easily!

Taste and smell

Be aware that excessive intake of salty foods and a craving for salty foods indicate a shortage of Nat. Mur. Very often, people sprinkle salt over food before tasting it. This sprinkled salt is too coarse to be absorbed by the body, and may raise the blood pressure. The 'cola-and-chips' syndrome is becoming prevalent, not only among youngsters but among the elderly as well. The combination of sweet carbonated drinks and salty foods gives a sugar overload and weakens the bones, which we cannot afford at any time of our lives, but especially not as we age. In cases where the sense of taste and smell have been compromised, take two tablets each of Nat. Mur. and Kali. Sulph. frequently throughout the day.

The digestive system

Remember that Nat. Mur. plays a major role in the digestive process. Minute sodium chloride particles separate in the peptic glands (ulcers can begin in these glands when there is too little Nat. Mur.). Metabolism takes place, and sodium and carbonic acid enter the bloodstream as sodium carbonate. The chlorine dissolves into hydrochloric acid, which is an important processor of the food we swallow. Without hydrochloric acid we cannot digest food, and heartburn, bloating, indigestion, colic, burping and flatulence occur. Dissolve two Nat. Mur. tablets in the mouth every 10 minutes to correct this and relieve the discomfort, but be exact and persistent and sip a hot Nat. Mur. drink if necessary. To make the drink, dissolve 10 Nat. Mur. tablets in half a cup of hot water and sip slowly (hold the fluid in the mouth so it mixes with the saliva) and remember to avoid table salt for a while!

It is interesting to note that coarse, non-iodised sea salt and pink Himalayan salt crystals do not have the same composition as table salt and are altogether more 'sympathetic' to the digestive system.

Together with digestive problems, constipation can be a real concern. When the stools are hard, dry and impacted, mashed papaya or pawpaw comes to the rescue with plain Bulgarian or Greek yoghurt to reinstate the correct bacteria in the gut. Figs (fresh or dried) also ease constipation, even chronic constipation, and soothe dry cracks around the anus. Drink a Nat. Mur. hot drink (10 tablets dissolved in half a cup of hot water), eat half a cup of plain Bulgarian yoghurt with half a cup of dried soaked prunes or figs, and feel the difference. The entire digestive process eases and becomes healthy. Buy dried figs when fresh figs are not in season and soak them overnight in warm water in which 10 Nat. Mur. tablets have been dissolved.

Nausea, vertigo, a bloated feeling and watery diarrhoea all benefit from two Nat. Mur. tablets sucked frequently until the condition passes and the system reverts to normal. I have found that Nat. Mur. (included in the colic formula 7, 8, 9, 10 and 11) works very well for any of the above digestive ailments. It handles both diarrhoea and constipation and is a soothing corrective remedy worth considering.

The urinary system

Elderly people often have to make frequent trips to the toilet, and there can be a weak flow of urine. When the trips are irritatingly frequent and create a feeling of desperation, Nat. Mur. is indicated. Suck two tablets 4–8 times through the day and leave a bottle of Nat. Mur. in the bathroom to remind you to suck two tablets every time you go there!

Dehydration and sunstroke

If you become dehydrated, especially in hot weather, frequent Nat. Mur. will soon restore the correct balance to the body. In the case of sunstroke, suck two Nat. Mur. tablets every 10 minutes, use wet towels to cool the system and call the doctor immediately. In very hot weather and when you find yourself perspiring continuously, dissolve 10 Nat. Mur. tablets in half a glass of cold water and sip frequently. Remember to give the same drink to overheated children and to your panting dog!

The circulatory system

Hands and feet can become cold in the ageing years, but equally, older people feel the heat more intensely too. Nat. Mur. will help to improve the circulation and steady the sense of heat and cold, and it is especially useful to relieve blue hands and feet. I add Nat. Mur. tablets to the hand and foot creams I make to ease any discomfort in the extremities, and Nat. Mur. cream is exceptionally soothing for haemorrhoids and varicose veins too.

Nat. Mur. circulation cream

1½ cups good aqueous cream
1 cup pennywort leaves (*Centella asiatica*)
1 cup chopped comfrey (*Symphytum officinale*) leaves
½ cup celery seeds, flowers and tops of the stems
2 tablespoons olive oil
2 tablespoons baobab oil
4 teaspoons vitamin E oil
10 Nat. Mur. tablets dissolved in a tablespoon of hot water

Simmer the aqueous cream, pennywort, comfrey and celery together in a double boiler for 20 minutes. Keep pressing the herbs down well and stir frequently. Strain through a fine sieve and add the olive, baobab and vitamin E oils. Mix thoroughly. Add the dissolved Nat. Mur. tablets and mix again. Spoon the cream into screw-top glass jars, label and store in the fridge. When you want to use it as a massage cream, warm the jar by standing it in hot water.

This circulation cream can be used to massage the back, and it can be smoothed over the feet, hands and neck. It is also helpful when there is congestion, fever blisters and head colds. Never underestimate the power of a healing cream in sympathetic hands, including for emotional conditions such as grief and feelings of isolation.

Female problems

As women enter menopause and beyond there can be uterine cramps, dips into depression, sadness and anxiety, decrease in libido, and headaches. During this time, Nat. Mur. does a wonderful balancing act and should be taken together with Ferrum Phos., Kali. Sulph., Mag. Phos. and Silica to help ease the menopause transition. It can also be combined with Calc. Phos. and Silica for osteoporosis, which can take us unawares after menopause.

How you feel

Nat. Mur. has the exceptional ability to lift the spirits and to lighten negative tendencies ranging from bad temper, blaming others and road rage, to anxiety, insecurity, gloominess, indifference, 'nit-picking', impatience and dwelling on past grievances. All such moods call for Nat. Mur. and will benefit from it daily. Suck two Nat. Mur. tablets six times a day, reduce your sugar intake, and include Nat. Mur.-rich vegetables and fruits in the diet. A positive change will begin and bring a turnaround.

Nat. Mur. is often deficient in the elderly and thus many of the above emotions can manifest. To start the day well, make a hot Nat. Mur. drink first thing in the morning, especially in the face of anxiety and uncertainty. I would like to be remembered as a happy, loving grandmother and as a positive, grateful and helpful old person, so Nat. Mur. is part of my daily tissue salt intake! Dissolve 10 Nat. Mur. tablets in half a cup of hot water, stir thoroughly and sip slowly to start a great day!

Other ailments

The following conditions and symptoms all call for Nat. Mur.: allergic rhinitis, hay fever, endocrine imbalance, diabetes, limb-jerking during sleep, asthma, insomnia, sinusitis, irregular heartbeat, debility and lack of energy, swollen legs and ankles, hair loss (alopecia), joints that crack audibly, chronic stiffness, burning piles, chronic syphilis or gonorrhoea, arthritic pains and swellings, low or poor immunity, warts of all kinds, tearfulness and grief, gastroenteritis, diarrhoea, repetitive sneezing, constant thirst (often linked to diabetes), heavy sweating, hot stuffy itchy ears caused by an allergic reaction, and overindulgence in alcohol.

If you are experiencing anything on this list, top up on Nat. Mur.! The list applies to so many of us who are ageing; in fact, I have not yet found anyone aged over 50 who does not have a few of these symptoms, which means that Nat. Mur. tablets and Nat. Mur. foods should be a part of our everyday regimen. As an elderly lecturer, I keep a bottle always on hand – Nat. Mur. helps me 'keep my cool', as the students say!

Secondary and complementary tissue salts

Several tissue salts work well with Nat. Mur., namely Ferrum Phos., Nat. Phos., Kali. Phos., Calc. Phos. and Silica. A combination of all six makes a superb tonic, which I make frequently. I love the strong positive vibe it leaves me with, and notice that with this formula as a 'turbo-boost', I can keep on keeping on! To make the warm drink, crush 6–10 tablets each of Nat. Mur., Ferrum Phos., Nat. Phos., Kali. Phos., Calc. Phos. and Silica in a cup of hot water. Stir well until all are dissolved and sip slowly. The same drink can be made with cold water on a hot day.

Nat. Mur. herbal 'salt'

One of the easiest and most tasty ways to include some of these delicious herbs in the diet is to make a Nat. Mur. 'salt'. This versatile flavouring is sodium-free and is great ground over food as a substitute for table salt.

1 cup thyme leaves
1 cup mustard leaves
1 cup parsley leaves
1 cup oregano leaves
1 cup marjoram sprigs
1 cup celery leaves, seeds and flowers
1 cup sesame seeds
1 cup mustard seeds

Pick one cup of each herb (or one tablespoon if you prefer to make a smaller quantity at a time). Dry the herbs on sheets of brown paper in the shade, shaking them daily until they are dry. Once they have dried, strip the leaves from the stalks and crush them. Add a cup (or tablespoon depending on which measurement you used for the herb mix) of sesame seeds and mustard seeds and stir in well. This mix is superb used as food flavouring and can replace a lot of salt. (Remember to use coarse sea salt, non-iodised salt or ground Himalayan salt and not fine white table salt!)

Herbs that contain Nat. Mur.

Nat. Mur. herbs are deliciously versatile and fairly easy to grow. Try planting the following flavour-filled healing herbs at your kitchen door so that you have them on hand for daily use: comfrey, borage, calendula, chickweed, celery, thyme, oregano, marjoram, garden violets and chamomile (for further information on these herbs see *My 100 Favourite Herbs*).

Borage (*Borago officinalis*): This beautiful, rich, oily herb is excellent for dry skin conditions, such as eczema, as well as varicose veins, sprains, and kidney and bladder infections. Borage is an easy-to-grow annual and the leaves and flowers are delicious in soups and stews.

Buckwheat (*Fagopyrum esculentum*): Buckwheat is easy to grow and can be enjoyed as a green salad leaf, flower and sprout. It is a valuable health booster, and is good for circulation.

Calendula (*Calendula officinalis*): Calendula is a winter annual that eases skin irritations, grazes, burns and scratches. It is wonderful in a skin cream, as a cleansing lotion and in food.

Celery (*Apium graveolens*): An excellent detoxifier that clears toxins from the blood and the liver, and flushes the kidney and bladder.

Chamomile (*Chamomilla recutita*): A calming, soothing herb that also has a detoxifying effect.

Chickweed (*Stellaria media*): This cold-weather weed, which is commonly found in gardens, is excellent for rashes, grazes, skin ailments, chest infections, rheumatic pains, and inflammatory conditions like ulcers, boils and eczemas.

Comfrey (*Symphytum officinale*): A wonderful herb for treating arthritis, wounds, slow healing, skin conditions and chest ailments. Comfrey is rich in Nat. Mur. and makes a soothing cream and wash.

Garden violets (*Viola odorata*): This is a plant we should all grow for clearing congestion. It is excellent as a tea for coughs and colds, headaches, flu, bronchitis – as it helps to clear mucus.

Mustard (*Brassica nigra*): The fresh leaves and flowers should be included in our daily salads. Mustard is rich in minerals – especially iron – and is also good for clearing coughs and chestiness.

Oregano (*Origanum vulgarus*): Oregano makes a wonderful food flavouring and is also valuable as a heart-protection antioxidant and anti-inflammatory.

Thyme (*Thymus* species): A wonderful antiseptic herb that is rich is several tissue salts, and it is important to add thyme fresh to savoury dishes.

To make tea using any of the above herbs, pour a cup of boiling water over ¼ cup fresh herbs and allow it to draw for five minutes. Stir the tea well, then strain and add 10 crushed Nat. Mur. tablets and sip slowly. Herb teas are delicious and naturally healing (you will find many different recipes in my herbal tea book, titled simply *Tea*).

Foods rich in Nat. Mur.

Nat. Mur. is abundant in seafood; however, allergic reactions to seafood can occur in some people. Steamed white fish is easy and if you enjoy fish, include it in the diet twice-weekly. Avoid fried foods and tempting take-away foods. Remember that monosodium glutamate (MSG) is used as a flavouring in many take-away foods and can trigger allergic reactions such as hay fever, wheezing and asthma. Rather use the safe Nat. Mur. 'salt' in the recipe on p.96.

Lentil (magic) salad

2 cups brown lentils
1 cup split peas
2 litres water or good stock
2 large onions, chopped
3 tablespoons olive oil
Juice of 1 lemon
1–2 tablespoons mild curry powder
2 tablespoons chopped fresh thyme
3 tablespoons chopped celery
2 tablespoons chopped parsley
1–2 teaspoons Himalayan salt
2 teaspoons crushed coriander seeds
2 tablespoons coriander leaves

Simmer the lentils and split peas in water until tender, then drain. Fry the onions in the olive oil until they start to brown. Add this to the cooked lentils and split peas with all the other ingredients. I mix the curry powder with the lemon juice and a touch of water first before adding it. Use more curry powder if you prefer a spicier dish. Warm everything together in a steamer and serve hot with grilled fish, lean grilled beef or lean organic Karoo mutton. The coriander in this dish helps clear heavy metals from the body.

Beef and mutton are also rich in Nat. Mur., and can be used in healthy stews and stir-fries. Cabbage, spinach, asparagus, beetroot, carrot, lentils, radish, tomatoes and peas are all rich in Nat. Mur., as are almonds, walnuts, sesame seeds, figs (fresh and dried), apples and strawberries. Sumptuous juices, smoothies and soups can be made with these living foods, and it is worth growing as many of them as you can.

One of my favourite juices is my 'Nat. Mur. anti-ageing juice' (see p.100). I make it frequently, as it is so rich in vitality-boosting ingredients. Think of it as a tonic super food and make it fresh every time, as that is the way to get the best benefit from it.

Nat. Mur. stew

SERVES 6

This stew is a favourite and can be varied with the vegetables in season. It is worth making weekly, as it keeps well in the fridge and can be frozen.

Olive oil
2 or 3 large onions, chopped
1 or 2 mutton loin chops per person, or good stewing mutton or beef
4 carrots, sliced
2 cups celery, chopped roughly
1 cup brown lentils
4–6 medium-sized sweet potatoes, scrubbed and cut into wedges
2–4 well-chopped tomatoes
Fresh thyme or oregano
Juice of 1 or 2 lemons
Himalayan salt and cayenne pepper to taste

Pour a little olive oil into a heavy-bottomed pot. Brown the onions and then the meat, stirring frequently. Add the remaining ingredients and enough water to cover. Simmer until tender, checking frequently, and turn down the heat so that the stew cooks slowly. Once the meat is tender, remove from the stove and keep covered. Serve the stew hot, sprinkled with chopped fresh parsley, together with brown rice, lemon wedges and steamed green peas.

Nat. Mur. anti-ageing juice

SERVES 1

2 stalks fresh parsley
2 carrots, peeled
2 apples, peeled and cored
2 beetroots, peeled and quartered
2 cups wheatgrass sprouts or young micro-greens
½ a fresh pineapple, peeled and cubed
1–2 cups buckwheat greens

Press all the ingredients through a juicer. Drink the juice immediately.
Barley sprouts and grass, young radish plants and beetroot leaves can all
be added. It is worth growing sprouts and micro-greens, such as wheat,
barley, buckwheat, radish, parsley, mung beans, lucerne, sunflowers,
peas, lentils, sesame seeds, beetroot and celery to include in this
wonderful juice, as they confer so much energy and vitality. The Herbal
Centre posts seeds and information countrywide as we are dedicated to
sprouting and micro-greens.

10 Nat. Phos.

Phosphate of Soda • *Natrum Phosphoricum*

Nat. Phos. is the antacid of the biochemic world, and its role in neutralising acids in the body is a remarkable one. We cannot manage without Nat. Phos., as it is the tissue salt that protects us from many ailments. I have found it to be one of the most consistently used tissue salts as acidity is so much in evidence today.

The fluids within the body contain acids as well as alkalis. Acidity is therefore always present in the blood, muscles, brain cells, nerves and in the inter-cellular fluid. When the body becomes too acidic, the system will respond quickly to Nat. Phos. Suck two tablets every 10–15 minutes until the tension resolves.

It is absolutely necessary that an equilibrium be maintained between acid and alkaline in the body, and that the balance of Calc. Phos. is in harmony with Nat. Phos. so that protein can be absorbed into the bones, tendons and joints in the correct amounts. Nat. Phos. helps maintain the perfect ratio between acid and alkaline, which is vitally important to our health.

For example, Nat. Phos. keeps uric acid soluble in the blood, as this acid otherwise combines with any carbonic acid present and results in acidity being deposited in the joints, which causes pain and discomfort. Nat. Phos. also aids in the assimilation of fats and prevents thickening or viscosity in the bile and bile duct. All this indicates how tremendously important it is to eat the 'antacids' or Nat. Phos.-rich foods, and to include extra Nat. Phos. tissue salts in our daily regimen in order to maintain that wonderful state of high-level wellness!

Nat. Phos. also breaks down lactic acid into carbonic acid and water within the body; if it were not broken up, this acid would decompose or catalyse and irritate the tissues to the extent of causing pain, stiffness and discomfort. Nat. Phos. keeps carbonic acid in the lungs until it is exhaled, and in so doing reduces build-up in the body, as lactic acid can accumulate quickly, causing fatigue and stiffness (even brisk walking can do this). Thus we cannot afford to be without this tissue salt, especially as the years add up, bringing increasing stiffness.

10 Nat. Phos.

The skeleton

I pay great attention to Nat. Phos. when there is weakness in the legs, aching joints and gout. The entire skeleton benefits from a hot Nat. Phos. drink, made by dissolving 10 tablets each of Nat. Phos. and Ferrum Phos. in a glass of hot water. Sip the drink slowly to ease the pain of arthritis and gout, as well as aching joints and weakness in the legs.

A herb I have written about recently, ashwagandha (*Withania somnifera*), makes a particularly comforting tea for these conditions, with five tablets each of Nat. Phos., Nat. Sulph. and Silica dissolved in it. To make the tea, pour a cup of boiling water over ¼–½ cup ashwagandha leaves, berries and twigs. Stir well for five minutes, then strain. Add the crushed tissue salts or half a teaspoon each of the tissue salt powders, stir well and sip slowly. The secret is to hold the tea in the mouth as long as possible.

For many years I have made a soothing cream for aching joints, arthritic shoulders, and back and hip problems. I still make this cream today and post it countrywide. It includes two excellent herbs for pain, namely comfrey and pennywort.

The skin

Rashes, heat bumps, itchiness of the anus, shins, ankles, and between the fingers and toes, all respond to extra Nat. Phos. Take the tissue salt several times a day and make a Nat. Phos. spritz-spray, as it is a remarkable soother. To prepare it, dissolve 10 tablets each of Nat. Phos. and Ferrum Phos. in two cups of warm boiled water, or stir in one level teaspoon of Nat. Phos. powder, which we post countrywide. Pour into a spritz-spray bottle and shake well to disperse the tissue salts. Spray frequently over the hot, itchy rash or make a paste with 10 crushed tissue salts (or one teaspoon of the powder) and a little warm boiled water to spread over the area. Repeat as necessary.

If your scalp feels itchy, add Nat. Phos. to the conditioner after shampooing and feel the difference. Mix 10 crushed Nat. Phos. tablets or one teaspoon of Nat. Phos. powder into a cup of conditioner and give the mixture a few minutes to work on the scalp and hair. Then rinse off with warm water (a dash of apple cider vinegar can be added to the final rinse).

Nat. Phos. is one of the most valuable beauty treatments I know, and I have lectured on its use at beauty schools for many years. Nat. Phos. combined with Calc. Phos. and Kali. Sulph., together with herbs like pennywort and borage, can actually produce new skin cells. Try the remarkable anti-ageing cream on p.104, which can be posted countrywide.

The same tissue salts and herbs can be made into a spritz-spray and used on the face twice daily after washing; this will act as a tonic for the skin. Continue to take two tablets of each of the three tissue salts orally two or three times a day to encourage skin regeneration. As we age, this cream becomes more and more vital.

Soothing arthritis cream

1½ cups good aqueous cream
1 cup chopped fresh comfrey leaves (*Symphytum officinale*)
1 cup chopped pennywort leaves (*Centella asiatica*)
3 teaspoons vitamin E oil
2 teaspoons rose pelargonium oil
10 tablets each of Nat. Phos., Nat. Sulph. and Silica, finely crushed

Simmer the aqueous cream, comfrey and pennywort in a double boiler for 20 minutes, pressing the herbs down thoroughly in the cream and against the sides of the pot to release the precious healing oils. (Use of comfrey externally is considered safe, but comfrey tea taken internally is said to affect the liver, and doctors warn against it.) After 20 minutes, remove the pot from the heat and allow it to cool for 10 minutes. Strain out the leaves (tie them in a piece of muslin and use in the bath over stiff sore joints, then discard). Add the vitamin E and rose pelargonium oils and mix well.

The vitamin E oil helps to preserve the cream and the rose pelargonium helps the muscles to relax, and also has a beautiful fragrance. Finally, add the finely crushed tissue salt tablets. This little trio helps to ease stiffness, pain and discomfort. Or use one teaspoon each of the tissue salts in powder form and mix in well.

Always warm the cream before using it (stand the jar in a bowl of hot water) and massage it in gently and steadily. This helps to soothe away the soreness of chronic arthritis, rheumatism and gout – and remember gout is not only felt in the big toe! Certain foods must be avoided during a gout attack and when there is arthritis. Become familiar with these, as well as with the herbs and tissue salts that ease these conditions, as in this way you can control a great deal of discomfort and pain.

Anti-ageing Nat. Phos. cream

2 cups good aqueous cream
1 cup fresh pennywort (*Centella asiatica*) leaves, finely chopped
1 cup borage (*Borago officinalis*) leaves, flowers and stems, finely chopped
10 tablets each of Calc. Phos., Kali. Sulph. and Nat. Phos., crushed
3 teaspoons vitamin E oil
1–2 teaspoons neroli (or rose-scented pelargonium or lavender) essential oil
1 tablespoon avocado oil (in winter)

Simmer the aqueous cream, pennywort and borage in a double boiler for 30 minutes. Press the herbs down to release the oils and stir frequently. Remove from the heat and let the mixture cool for about an hour. Press through a new strainer into a glass bowl. Add the finely crushed tissue salts and stir thoroughly. Finally, mix in the vitamin E oil and the essential oil. In winter, add the avocado oil. Spoon into sterilised glass jars with good lids and label. This will become your most loved cream for the face, hands, legs and heels! Store excess in the fridge.

The head

A headache on the crown or in the forehead region with throbbing almost dizzying pain, often upon waking in the morning, and with a creamy deposit on the back of the tongue, indicates a Nat. Phos. deficiency. Ferrum Phos. may also be deficient if there is intense pressure and even heat around the head. Suck two Nat. Phos. tablets every 5–10 minutes until the symptoms ease. Or dissolve 10 tablets each of Nat. Phos. and Ferrum Phos. in a cup of hot water and sip slowly. This will also ease gastric symptoms, such as sour belching and diarrhoea, that may occur with the headache.

The eyes

Conjunctivitis (red, itchy, tired eyes that are glued together in the morning by a thick, creamy-yellow discharge) indicates a lack of Nat. Phos. and high acidity in the body. A hot 'tea' can be made using 10 tablets each of Nat. Phos. and Ferrum Phos., crushed and dissolved in a cup of hot water. Allow the brew to cool to a comfortable temperature, then soak pads of cotton wool in it and use as a lotion to clear the discharge and soothe the eyes.

The ears

When the ears are hot, itchy and uncomfortable, or if the outer ear feels sore, sometimes with a burning feeling and gastric disturbance, suck two Nat. Phos. tablets alternately with two Ferrum Phos. tablets. This will quickly soothe the discomfort.

Oral health

Restless sleep and teeth grinding at night indicate a lack of Nat. Phos. Two Nat. Phos. tablets sucked at intervals through the day, and at night, will lead to a marked improvement. When teeth grinding is accompanied by an itchy anus, consult your doctor in case of parasite infection.

The digestive system

We tend to forget how vital digestion is to good health. However, if any of the following symptoms affect you, then Nat. Phos. is likely to be deficient in your body and the tissue salt treatment should be part of your daily routine.

- A feeling of heat and discomfort or 'churning' in the stomach and intestines.
- A dislike of once favourite foods, and not feeling satisfied after a meal.
- Constantly searching the fridge or grocery cupboards for something tasty to eat.
- Sour reflux, belching, burping of sour gas, and a yellowish coating on the back of the tongue.
- Occasional vomiting of sour foods.
- Repeated heartburn.
- Repeated discomfort, dyspepsia, stomach ulcers, stools that leave a burning discomfort, or if there is sour-smelling diarrhoea, possibly even worms.

These symptoms are all indications that Nat. Phos. is seriously deficient. Start by sucking two Nat. Phos. tablets before and after eating. Keep a glass of water nearby (always boil the water first and cool) into which 10 Nat. Phos. tablets have been dissolved, and take frequent sips.

Nat. Phos. helps to ease food allergies, as it assists the body to adapt. It is worth trying the tissue salt and keeping notes to record your progress. Remember, start first by sucking two Nat. Phos. tablets at intervals, or sip a glass of water into which 6–10 Nat. Phos. tablets have been dissolved.

10 Nat. Phos.

A headache with sour vomiting and belching responds quickly to Nat. Phos. and Nat. Sulph. together. Nausea can be stilled by sucking two Nat. Phos. tablets and this will also ease liver discomfort. In the case of jaundice, where there is yellowness of the skin and the whites of the eyes, suck two Nat. Phos. tablets frequently and consult your doctor. Do not try to treat jaundice on your own.

The urinary system

If urine is released when coughing or sneezing, or there is an inability to hold the urine, this can be helped by sucking two Nat. Phos. tablets three or four times a day. You can also use a very comforting formula, namely two tablets each of Nat. Phos., Calc. Phos., Kali. Phos. and Nat. Mur., taken 4–6 times a day. Do bladder exercises at the same time, as this will strengthen the bladder amazingly. To tighten the pelvic floor, cross the legs while standing, press the knees and thighs together and pull up the pelvic floor. Hold for a count of 10, then release; repeat 10 times and do this exercise 10 times a day. This will begin to re-educate the sphincter at the base of the bladder and strengthen it. Nat. Phos. supports us beautifully in accomplishing this!

Female problems

As women age, chronic cystitis can occur and cause much discomfort. There is often excessive vaginal excretion and an accompanying itch, redness and burning distress. All indicate the need for Nat. Phos. Suck two tablets 4–8 times through the day, as this will greatly relieve the condition, and use the tissue salts in a wash every time you go to the toilet.

To make the tissue salt wash, dissolve 10 crushed tablets each of Nat. Phos. and Ferrum Phos. in a bowl containing two litres of warm water. Very gently rinse away any urine or discharge. Use a clean cloth each time, and wash or wipe the area over a toilet or bidet. Keep the bowl covered when not in use.

A gentle Nat. Phos. douche also helps to clear the discharge and is very easy to make. Dissolve 10 crushed Nat. Phos. tablets (or 1 teaspoon of powder) in a litre of warm water together with half a cup of apple cider vinegar, mix thoroughly and use once at night for three consecutive evenings. Make a fresh douche daily.

Dust the area with talcum powder containing Nat. Phos. (we post a rice-flour talcum powder containing Nat. Phos. countrywide). The talcum powder does not contain any fragrance or additives. It is tremendously soothing and freshening and helps to control the discharge and the itch; it also helps with itching and sweating in the underarm area.

When there is frequent urination, inability to retain urine, and acidity, which could correspond with rheumatism and with a sour smell, go onto Nat. Phos. daily for at least three months. Suck two tablets two or three times a day or make a hot drink with 10 crushed tablets in a glass of warm water. Add 10 Ferrum Phos. tablets if there is pain and inflammation, and sip it frequently through the day.

How you feel

When the body becomes acidic, 'acid' emotions such as anger, irritability, vindictiveness, bullying, competitiveness, selfishness, envy and conflict gain power. Nat. Phos. works well here too, so be sure to keep a good supply of this wonderful antacid tissue salt.

Other ailments

All the symptoms and conditions below indicate a lack of Nat. Phos., although we tend to overlook them in our busy lives. I have added to this list over the years and have been astonished at how quickly Nat. Phos. works!

If you awaken with a feeling of nausea and dizziness, almost unable to lift your head for fear of falling, or if you cannot find your balance, suck two tablets every half hour for the next three or four hours. Start with four tablets initially, followed by two more every 15 minutes for an hour to release the tension. Then follow with two tablets half-hourly.

Palpitations and irregular heart action can be caused by the digestive system. When this is accompanied by shakiness or trembling after eating sip a Nat. Phos. hot drink (10 tablets or one teaspoon of Nat. Phos. powder dissolved in a cup of hot water). The trembling and palpitations should lessen quite quickly once Nat. Phos. is in the system. Whenever in doubt, consult your doctor immediately.

In the case of a blotchy red face (without a fever), with a pale area around the nose and mouth, and when there is rash-type blotchiness, suck two Nat. Phos. tablets every 30 minutes, three or four times. This will clear the congestion. Nose picking and fiddling with the nose also indicate a Nat. Phos. deficiency. Become aware of this habit.

To relieve sour-smelling perspiration with a fever, vomiting and headache, suck two Nat. Phos. tablets every 15 minutes until a doctor can be reached. When there is diarrhoea, include Nat. Phos. at least six times a day – the acidic smell will indicate a shortage of Nat. Phos.

10 | Nat. Phos.

Nat. Phos. in a non-lactose base is considered the best tissue salt for diabetes. If taken diligently every day, there is often a positive impact on the amount of insulin needed. However, this must be monitored by your doctor. Hypoglycaemia can be eased by increasing Nat. Phos. intake to at least six times a day, and sugar cravings will lessen with Nat. Phos.-rich foods and Nat. Phos. tablets taken at least four times daily.

Adult acne can occur, especially around middle age, with a rash over the nose, blackheads and an oily appearance to the skin. This indicates the need for additional Nat. Phos. and a Nat. Phos. wash at least three times a day.

Interestingly, tests done in Germany many years ago found that Nat. Phos. was remarkably helpful to morphine addicts in extreme pain. A small dose was administered by the doctor as a daily injection just under the skin, and the dose was increased as the need for the painkilling abilities of morphine lessened. Within three months the patients were cured.

Signs of Nat. Phos. deficiency

The old Swiss doctor who taught me the wonders of tissue salts often said that where there is a candida tendency, there will always be shortage of Nat. Phos. He said other signs are a red nose, spotty skin, hanging cheeks, a strong double chin in the elderly, and arthritic and rheumatic aches and pains.

Secondary and complementary tissue salts

Nat. Sulph. is an excellent working partner with Nat. Phos.; however, the strength of Nat. Phos. enhances the workings of all the tissue salts. Something to remember is that Nat. Phos. combined with Calc. Phos. and Mag. Phos. will maintain an excellent acid-alkaline balance in the body – these three show immediate results. They are very important in balancing us and maintaining good energy and vitality, and serve as an anti-ager for the 50-year-old as much as for the 80-year-old!

Herbs rich in Nat. Phos.

Aniseed (*Pimpinella anisum*): A valuable annual that aids the digestion, and helps to ease insomnia, spasmodic coughing, bronchitis, asthma, pneumonia, menstrual cycles, and even epileptic attacks. It has an excellent pain-relieving and tension-relaxing action. It makes an excellent tea.

Basil (*Ocimum basilicum*): This deliciously flavoured herb is a reliable expectorant and digestive, and treats coughs, colds and tension equally well. Basil tea is good for easing diarrhoea, dysentery and anxiety. No garden should be without basil – all the species have the same benefits.

Caraway (*Carum carvi*): A digestive herb that is an excellent diuretic, and helps with cramps, including menstrual pains, coughs and bruising.

Celery (*Apium graveolens*): The plant and seeds are excellent for clearing toxins, easing chest ailments, urinary problems, working on both the kidneys and bladder, lowering high blood pressure, and disposing of urates that cause stiffness and pain in the joints.

Coriander (*Coriandrum sativum*): This easy-to-grow annual is excellent for digestion, nervous tension, temper tantrums and bad moods. Make it into a tea, or crush and grind it over food.

Cumin (*Cuminum cyminum*): The seeds, fresh leaves and flowers are great for circulation, digestive ailments, especially flatulence, fever, feverish colds and stuffy noses, and for removing toxins from the body.

Dill (*Anthemum graveolens*): Dill sweetens the breath and eases hiatus hernia, colic, indigestion, hiccups, diverticulitis and digestive infections with colic, flatulence and bloating.

Fennel (*Foeniculum vulgare*): This is one of the best herbal detoxifiers and the much respected 'slimmer's herb'. Fennel also works for spotty skin, dry skin, constipation, colic and respiratory ailments. Chewing fennel seeds eases digestion.

Ginger (*Zingiber officinal*): This is a superb herb for respiratory ailments, nausea, travel sickness, nausea associated with chemotherapy, colic and digestive upsets. It combines well with honey as a cough mixture, makes a comforting tea and works as a circulatory herb that benefits cold hands and feet.

Lemon balm (*Melisa officianalis*): The most beautiful calming, relaxing unwinding, anti-colic, digestive herb we know. It helps with high blood pressure, muscular aches, shingles, chickenpox and anxiety, and has antibacterial, antiviral and antifungal properties. A vital herb with many uses, lemon balm also unwinds us and helps us sleep.

Lucerne/Alfalfa (*Medicago sativa*): Include fresh leaves and flowers in the diet and in teas for fatigue and menopause, and to strengthen the immune system for fighting coughs, colds and 'flu, especially as we age. Make a tea of lucerne with winter savoury (*Satureja montana*) as a tonic. Include fresh lucerne leaves in daily salads and stir-fries. Grow it as a sturdy perennial next to the kitchen for quick pickings.

Mint (*Mentha* species): There are many mints and all of them have the same digestive easing and relaxing qualities. Mint tea will ease headaches, migraines and feverish conditions. Peppermint tea is a trusted brain herb used during exams, it unblocks sinuses, acts as an antispasmodic and prevents vomiting.

Parsley (*Petroselium crispum*): One of nature's best detoxifiers and possibly the world's favourite herb, parsley is a powerhouse that helps with fever, nausea, liver problems, high blood pressure and bladder infections. Paired with garlic, it will help to lower high cholesterol.

Stinging nettle (*Urbica dioica*): A great cleanser and detoxifier, essential for gout, arthritis, kidney function, fluid retention, jaundice, catarrh, and an enlarged and painful prostate. Stinging nettle purifies the blood, treats anaemia, and soothes sciatica, bronchitis and catarrh.

Violet (*Viola odorata*): A gentle herb that treats headaches, coughs, colds, catarrh, hay fever, bronchitis, hangovers, blocked sinuses and sinus headaches, and is an excellent decongestant. It has also been used for tumours, both benign and cancerous. Violet tea is a true panacea. Use the leaves and the flowers.

To make a herb tea, pour a cup of boiling water over ¼ cup of any of the herbs mentioned above. Let the tea infuse for five minutes, stir well, strain and sip slowly. You can sweeten with a touch of honey or add a squeeze of lemon juice. Usually one cup of herbal tea a day is a good dose, but take it morning and evening if needed. Try chilling the herb teas in summer and serve them with a vegetable and fruit juice (see juice recipe p.111).

Digestive seed mix

Use this fabulous seed mix as a delicious sprinkle over all savoury dishes.

1 tablespoon each:
Fennel seeds
Coriander seeds
Caraway seeds
Aniseed
Dill seeds
Cumin seeds

Mix well and store the seeds in a glass screw-top jar. You can also put the seeds into a grinder, and grind this mix over all your meals. In this way you will get the digestive benefits of the seeds on a daily basis.

Nat. Phos. energy juice

SERVES 2

½ cup parsley
½ cup fresh lucerne
2 carrots, peeled
2 medium beetroots, peeled
2 medium apples, peeled and cored
1 cup strawberries or raspberries
½ a papaya, seeds and skin removed

Push the ingredients through a juicer and drink for a burst of energy!

Foods rich in Nat. Phos.

Nat. Phos. is present in an array of tasty foods and can be included in your diet effortlessly.

Foods that are rich in Nat. Phos. include: brown rice, lentils, beetroot, asparagus, carrots, corn, spinach, olives, oats, rosehips, plain Bulgarian yoghurt, grapes, raspberries, mulberries, strawberries, raisins, apples, peaches, apricots, pawpaw, quinces and watermelon.

For breakfast, have a bowl of oats with plain Bulgarian yoghurt, sesame seeds, a little grated fresh ginger, a grated apple and a few berries or fruit in season, and in winter add sundried raisins. Make smoothies, juices and fruit salads, and serve with sesame seeds and plain yoghurt. Grow New Zealand spinach and your own lentils for soups and stews.

Nat. Phos. smoothie

Many years ago I became known for a Nat. Phos. drink I loved making as a smoothie. I have always loved this refresher, which can be the energiser we often need in the heat of midsummer!

¼ cup sundried sultanas, soaked in hot water for an hour
2 sprigs lemon balm (Melissa)
1 cup fresh strawberries, sliced
1 cup plain Bulgarian yoghurt
2 cups sliced skinned peaches, apple or papaya (or all together)
2 slices fresh ginger
Pinch or two of cumin and coriander seeds
½ cup fresh parsley sprigs

Soak the sultanas in half a cup of water for 15 minutes. Soak the lemon balm in half a cup of boiling water for about 10 minutes. Put all the ingredients (including the water) in a blender and whirl until smooth. This smoothie is delicious and will set you up for the day, or for a busy afternoon if taken at lunchtime.

Detoxing with watermelon

Watermelon is wonderful for treating high acidity in the body, but must be taken on its own. It makes a refreshing, cleansing smoothie in the heat of midday or in the afternoon when you feel life is too rushed and pressured. Simply whirl four cups of watermelon pieces with their seeds in a blender – just that, nothing more. Don't eat anything after the watermelon smoothie for at least an hour. Water is fine, but do not ingest anything else. During the festive period, when one is inclined to overindulge, try to drink a watermelon smoothie once a week.

11 Nat. Sulph.

Sodium Sulphate • Sulphate of Soda •
Natrum Sulphuricum

Known as *sal mirabile*, 'the wonderful salt', Nat. Sulph. was one of the first salts to be developed by Dr Schuessler from the natural alkaline waters of Europe in the early 19th century. It has never lost its popularity, although we tend to neglect this remarkable salt today, even though we need it as a detoxifier and cleanser, living as we do in air-conditioned buildings and amid pollution. We also tend to forget its exceptional role as a liver support.

My first studies of Nat. Sulph. focused on its ability to regulate the density of intercellular fluids by removing toxins and excess water from the body. It is a waste remover and cell cleanser of note, helpful for diabetics and the elderly people with fluid on the lungs. Nat. Sulph. is essential to the health of the pancreas, intestines and the entire urinary system, and will help reduce obesity around the thighs. It can be taken long term with very helpful results.

As we age, Nat. Sulph. is a marvellous panacea, as it has a stimulating effect on the cell linings. Known as Glauber's salt when it is chemically manufactured, and as sodium sulphate in chemistry, it can be produced easily by the action of sulphuric acid on ordinary table salt. It occurs naturally in Russia's salt lakes, and is used in this natural form as a biochemic cell salt.

Depression can occur when there is chronic pain or a feeling of being overburdened with responsibilities, and thoughts of suicide can arise at these times. Here is where Nat. Sulph. brings relief, as well as a feeling of hope, and a reduced feeling of being burdened. Nat. Sulph. has been called 'the kind and helpful crutch', as it enables one to step forward again.

Arnica of the mind and emotions

Many ancient texts refer to Nat. Sulph. as the 'arnica of the mind and emotions'. Just as arnica is applied to heal physical aches, so Nat. Sulph. taken internally relieves many emotional symptoms, particularly during times of intense despair, grief, loss and adjustment.

The skin

Nat. Sulph. is needed for severe, overwhelming skin itchiness that is often triggered by changes in pressure, such as when undressing. Chafed areas, watery secretions, hot itchy irritated skin, eczema, rashes and crusty scabs all call for a Nat. Sulph. lotion and a dusting of cornflour, not scented talcum powder. For washing, use pure baby shampoo or soapwort wash.

Soapwort wash

2 cups soapwort (*Sapponaria officinalis*) leaves, sprigs and flowers
2 litres water

Simmer the soapwort in the water for 30 minutes, pressing the sprigs down frequently as it boils. Cool and strain. Use it as a warm and soothing wash over the area frequently. Make it fresh or store excess in the fridge.

Nat. Sulph. lotion

20 Nat. Sulph. tablets
10 tablets each of Nat. Phos. and Nat. Mur.
1½ cups warm water (that has been boiled)

Dissolve the tissue salts in the warm water. Store the lotion in a labelled spritz-spray bottle. Shake the lotion well before use. When it's cold, warm the lotion by standing the bottle in a jug of hot water – test carefully before applying. In hot weather it will cool mosquito bites. Dab it onto hard-to-reach places by soaking a cotton wool pad in the lotion and applying it to the area.

The skeleton

As we age we tend to feel aching pains in the lower back, hips, knees, ankles, shoulders and neck. The joints can feel stiff and out of alignment, and rheumatic pains can envelop us, often with cracking sounds, aggravated by humidity, cold or moisture in the air. Nat. Sulph. helps to keep the extremities warm, so suck two tablets frequently, especially before bed.

Old head injuries, dental problems, gout, sciatic pain down the back of the leg, and aching joints respond well to Nat. Sulph. These conditions can also be relieved with a hot Nat. Sulph. drink, sipped frequently.

The head

Use Nat. Sulph. for a nauseous headache verging on a migraine, with sour vomiting and a queasy stomach. Take two tablets each of Nat. Sulph. and Nat. Phos. every 10 minutes or until the symptoms disperse. When there is sluggishness in focusing the eyes, combined with a headache and a crusty yellow discharge at the corners of the eyes, Nat. Sulph. is vital. Suck two tablets every 10 minutes, or sip a hot Nat. Sulph. drink. To make it, dissolve 6–10 crushed tablets in ½–¾ cup of hot water, and sip slowly.

If there has been a bump to the head that causes a splitting headache, congestion or a feeling of fuzziness, sip the Nat. Sulph. drink above and see a doctor in case of traumatic brain injury. Add six drops of tea tree essential oil to two teaspoons of Nat. Sulph. 'tea' and mix well. Apply to the temples and under the nose to allow the tea tree to open the nose and ease the feeling of congestion and pressure.

The respiratory system

Nat. Sulph. eases a tight chest and difficult breathing, especially in damp, chilly weather. It is also a great comfort when there is asthma (combined with panic), wheezing, thick phlegm, and coughing up of yellow sputum. For coughing fits, sip a half cup of hot water with 6–10 tablets dissolved in it, as Nat. Sulph. can clear thick nasal discharge and heal mucous membranes.

An American specialist, Dr Charles Vaught, recommended that at the first signs of flu we should suck two Nat. Sulph. tablets every 15 minutes for two hours; then two tablets every half hour for the next three hours, and, finally, two tablets every hour until the symptoms ease. I have also come to rely on his wonderful flu formula, namely tissue salts 1, 4, 5, 9 and 11 (this formula has remained in my head over the 50-plus years that I have used tissue salts!). Dissolve 10 tablets of each salt (Calc. Fluor., Ferrum Phos., Kali. Mur., Nat. Mur. and Nat. Sulph.) in a cup of hot water and sip frequently.

The digestive system

Nat. Sulph. is a great comfort when there is burning indigestion. Suck two tablets frequently and also make a hot drink by dissolving 6–10 tablets in half a cup of hot water (boiled and cooled to a comfortable temperature) and sip slowly. This will soothe the gall bladder and liver.

11 Nat. Sulph.

When there is a bitter taste in the mouth and the breath smells, with a greyish-brown coating on the tongue, suck two Nat. Sulph. tablets every half hour. Take this dose when there is abdominal bloating with colic, discomfort with tight clothing, and vomiting of green bile. This will soon clear the problem, so keep a bottle near at hand.

Sometimes watery diarrhoea alternates with constipation and flatulence. In these cases sip a Nat. Sulph. drink made with 6–10 tablets dissolved in ½–¾ cup of hot water, often with Nat. Mur. or Nat. Phos., to ease symptoms.

Sugar consumption needs to be monitored as we age, as our bodies can show symptoms of overload, and diabetes is on the increase. Nat. Sulph. is helpful here as it stimulates the pancreas, and foods containing this tissue salt are extremely important as part of the diabetic diet.

Malaria

Malaria needs to be treated by a doctor; however, tissue salts offer invaluable support. Symptoms include chills, remittent fever and sweating. Nat. Sulph. is an important treatment for this disease as it helps to normalise excess water in the cells, and, together with Kali. Phos. and Ferrum Phos., it normalises the nervous system and also reduces fever. Nat. Sulph. also relieves the vertigo, dizziness, feeling of pressure around the heart and bitter taste in the mouth that can occur. Suck two tablets frequently, up to 10 times a day. Also, make a tissue salt drink by dissolving 10 tablets each of Nat. Sulph. and Ferrum Phos. in a cup of hot water. Sip it slowly every now and then.

Female problems

As women age, they sometimes experience genital itching and discharge that does not respond to ointments, lotions or washes. Dissolve 10–20 Nat. Sulph. tablets in three cups of hot water and add half a cup of apple cider vinegar to the mixture. Use this as a wash with a clean facecloth or as a lotion dabbed on with cotton wool pads, or spritz-spray it on as a warm lotion (stand the bottle in a jug of hot water to warm it before spraying it on).

How you feel

We often neglect this aspect of our daily life; however, I notice that I have become more aware of emotions as I grow older. Too many people feel alone, unloved and unappreciated. Feelings of discouragement, melancholia, fear and even dread can lead to thoughts of suicide. Nat. Sulph. is clearly indicated at these times, and if it is taken regularly along with the other tissue salts, especially Kali. Phos., this despair can be lifted and peace restored.

Panic attacks can occur in the elderly when there is a feeling of not being able to swallow. This will be relieved by sucking two tablets of the 12-in-one tissue salt (Combin 12), followed by a hot Nat. Sulph. and Kali. Phos. drink (10 tablets of each dissolved in a cup of hot water), sipped slowly, peacefully and quietly. This will also relieve feelings of hopelessness and depression.

Nat. Sulph. soothes abrupt behaviour, short temper, irritability and impatience. At the other end of the spectrum it also dissipates lassitude, the feeling that you are too weary to tackle a task hanging over you, and it helps to relieve the heavy, anxious dreams that can come with it.

Interestingly, many of these feelings can be alleviated by going out into the sun, and sleeping in a sun-filled room where there is no damp or mould on the walls and floors. If possible, one should avoid living near water, especially damp, marshy places. We all need warmth, sunlight, positive experiences, positive people and liver-cleansing foods!

Secondary and complementary tissue salts

Nat. Sulph.'s closest companion salt is Nat. Phos.; together they clear over-acidic, liverish conditions beautifully, while Nat. Mur. and Nat. Sulph. regulate the metabolism and water within the body. Nat. Sulph., Calc. Sulph. and Silica give an energy spark to a depleted body; Nat. Sulph. with Ferrum Phos. helps to raise very low blood pressure; and Nat. Sulph. with Kali. Sulph. clears athlete's foot.

The magical formula for lifting the spirits, dispersing dark thoughts and easing general suffering is Nat. Sulph., Kali. Phos. and Calc. Phos. together.

Herbs that contain Nat. Sulph.

Burdock (*Arctium lappa*): This herb is an excellent antirheumatic, diuretic, mild laxative and a natural antibiotic. Use it in soups and stews or make the giant leaves into a tea.

Cayenne pepper (*Capsicum frutescens*): Home-grown organic cayenne is a wonderful antibacterial as well as a circulatory stimulant, and it deep cleanses mucus from the body. Eat two or three fresh slices of the hot pepper on home-baked bread with a little olive oil at the end of a meal with a hot cup of parsley tea. This is an old Italian recipe I learned in Italy during a cold winter and it is delicious.

Celery (*Apium graveolens*): A general cleanser, celery flushes toxins from the kidneys and liver and is an excellent antirheumatic and a urinary antiseptic.

Horseradish (*Armoracia rusticana*): This herb is a natural treatment for urinary and respiratory tract ailments and infections. Grate the fresh root and mix it with hot honey and apple cider vinegar (one cup horseradish, ½ cup honey and ½ cup apple cider vinegar), store it in a glass bottle and keep it sealed in the fridge. Eat it as a condiment with roasts or spread it onto bread and serve with cheese. It clears the chest, stimulates circulation and is a diuretic. The leaves can be chopped into salads and stir-fries.

Parsley (*Petroselinum crispum*): Parsley is rich in Nat. Sulph. and has a diuretic, cleansing and tonic action. To make it into a tonic tea, pour a cup of boiling water over ¼ cup fresh parsley, stir thoroughly, let the tea stand for five minutes and sip slowly.

Foods rich in Nat. Sulph.

Here is a list of wonderful Nat. Sulph.-rich foods to choose from: lentils, oats, spinach, kale, broccoli, cabbage, cauliflower, onions, pumpkin, pumpkin flowers, vine tips, leaves and tendrils, leeks, spring onions, paprika, cayenne peppers, green peppers, beetroot and beetroot leaves, New Zealand spinach, Welsh onions and their leaves, cucumber, bananas and apples.

Apple and banana smoothie

SERVES 1

This smoothie is great for boosting energy in the middle of a busy day! I grow a lot of wheatgrass and barley grass, and a big handful added to this delicious blend seems to give great vitality. Wheatgrass is incredibly rich in all the tissue salts, so it acts as a tonic and is very sustaining.

1 banana, peeled
2 apples, peeled and cored
½ cup pecan nuts or walnuts
½ cup husked sunflower seeds
1 cup wheatgrass

Push one apple through the juice extractor with the wheatgrass. Add the banana with the nuts and sunflower seeds and then follow with the second apple. Drink the smoothie slowly, holding every mouthful in the mouth for six seconds before swallowing.

Nat. Sulph.-rich hotpot

SERVES 6–8

This is a tasty and health-boosting stew that can be varied according to what is in season. It is easy to make and stores well in the fridge if there are any leftovers. I love making it with a whole organic chicken.

1 organic chicken
½ cup olive oil
3 cups sliced leeks
4 cups chopped Welsh onion, leaves included
2 cups chopped celery leaves and stems
2 large green peppers
2–3 cups New Zealand spinach
10 kale leaves, stripped off their stems
1 small cabbage
4 cups peeled, chopped pumpkin
4 cups broccoli, broken into pieces
4 medium-sized sweet potatoes, sliced into rounds, skin left on
4 large paprikas, de-seeded and chopped
Juice of 2 lemons
6 sprigs fresh thyme
2 litres strong chicken stock
2 tablespoons crushed coriander seeds
1 tablespoon cumin seeds
Cayenne pepper and sea salt to taste
1 cup chopped parsley to garnish

Brown the chicken in the olive oil, then add the leeks and brown further. Add the remaining ingredients except the parsley and simmer until the chicken is tender. Slice the chicken on a serving platter, then ladle the vegetables and the delicious stock over it. Keep a separate jug of stock to add when needed. For variation, you can replace the chicken with 4–6 mutton chops and add mint to the pot too. It is beautifully sustaining, warming and filling, and everyone enjoys it!

12 Silica

Silicon Dioxide • Quartz • *Silicea*

Known by some as 'the surgeon of the human organism', Silica is found in our hair, skin, nails and the membrane covering the bone (the periosteum). There is also a trace of it inside the bone, as well as to an extent in the blood, nerve sheaths and mucous membranes.

Silica is composed of infinitely minute jagged particles that cleanse the tissues of decaying organic matter, such as pus. Like a lancet, it cuts a passage to the surface of the skin so that the pus can be expelled. It is a toxin eliminator, ridding the body of splinters, boils, abscesses and bad odours. Because it expels foreign matter from the body, it may lead to the rejection of plates, screws, metal implants and even breast implants – *but only if it is taken in very large quantities for a prolonged period of time* and if there is an infection around the area. A normal dosage, such as taking two Silica tablets twice daily, will not eliminate surgical implants from healthy tissue.

However, when in doubt, leave out; rather increase the foods in which Silica is found in order to get as much benefit as possible from this remarkable tissue salt, as it works as a deep-acting cleanser and eliminator. Remember that Silica is found in the hair, skin, nails and all bone surfaces, in fact in the entire skeletal system, head to toe. We cannot build good health without it, particularly as we age, and there are times when we need to supplement with tablets. Silica is also in the nerve sheaths, where it acts as a protector and insulator, so include it in your daily health-building habits.

The skeleton

Lack of Silica affects the bones and spine; the structure becomes weak, with curvature of the spine and skeletal aches. Silica comes to the rescue here and is helpful where one is affected by weak bones, lumbago, sciatica (pain down the back of the leg), poor posture, weariness and fatigue, aching swollen legs, and swelling and pain in the feet. All elderly people have an ongoing need for Silica for the aches and pains of age, ulcerations, inflammation, diseased and fragile bones, chronic arthritis and rheumatism, bone tumours, and even obstinate neuralgias.

A disturbing little breathless cough with a painful spine will be soothed by Silica. Do not underestimate it, as it is essential for the connective tissue of the brain, as well as the whole skeleton. Two or three doses of two tablets of Silica a day will bring a soothing calm.

When there is chronic osteoporosis, suck two tablets three or four times a day. Silica also works well to relieve chronic fatigue, synovitis, weak ankles, hard tumours and painful ankylosing spondylitis that affects the spine, causing stiffening. A massage over the area with our strong 'herbal heat cream', which has Silica-rich plants in it, is wonderfully soothing and we can post this countrywide.

Deep, warm massage is beneficial for people suffering from painful joints and spine – I treated many patients with this complaint during my years as a physiotherapist. Keep the area warm after the massage, using a hot-water bottle with fresh lavender sprigs placed between the bottle and its cover, and let the person rest for about 20 minutes. This is soothing, unwinding and very comfortable for every patient.

A good general treatment for skeletal issues is two tablets each of Silica, Nat. Phos. and Nat. Mur. sucked 2–4 times a day. Many people have found this to be a real panacea for skeletal pain and discomfort.

The skin

Blind spots or pimples, subcutaneous cysts, scars and thin fragile skin all benefit from two Silica tablets sucked at least six times daily and a consistent application of Silica cream (see recipe on p.124). Remember that Silica will help to clear warts on the skin and fungal infection of the nails. It will also help to resolve nail ridges, thickened nails, breaking or flaking nails, white spots in the nails, and the discomfort of ingrown toe nails and haemorrhoids. Make a paste using six Silica tablets crushed and dissolved with a little water and apply daily to the nails, leaving it on to dry. Ensure that there is abundant Silica-rich food in the diet, supplemented with tablets daily.

Sweating can also increase as we age, especially from the head and feet; however, with extra Silica this can be well controlled as it neutralises and clears offensive-smelling perspiration. I add crushed Silica to my home-made talcum powders in midsummer and have received enthusiastic appreciation from so many, especially the elderly who struggle with foot odour in closed shoes.

12 Silica

> ## Silica foot deodoriser
>
> 15 finely crushed Silica tablets
> 2 cups rice flour
> 10 drops tea tree essential oil
>
> Mix the ingredients together thoroughly. Store in a glass jar with a
> good lid and shake up well each time you use it in a talcum powder
> dispenser. Shake a little daily into the shoes as well.

The head

When there are headaches, throbbing temples, unsteadiness and vertigo, suck two tablets frequently, at least four times a day, and you will soon feel better able to cope. After a stroke, Silica is a tremendous help as it absorbs the haematoma. Suck two tablets every half hour or every 15 minutes until the fear and discomfort ease.

When there is dry hair and hair loss, Silica encourages new growth and repairs itchy spots or nodules on the scalp. Two tablets sucked slowly six times a day will alleviate these symptoms.

Silica for healthy hair

Silica builds up the texture of hair by strengthening the hair shaft and controlling split ends, and it improves the condition by stimulating the hair follicles. Crush 10 Silica tablets very finely to a powder and mix into your conditioner. Work it into the scalp each time you wash your hair to keep the scalp in good health, and suck two Silica tablets at least twice a day to promote a thick, strong growth of hair.

The eyes

Often as we age, our eyes appear sunken and deep. There may also be red eyelids, styes or itching, with involuntary twitching or frequent blinking. Silica also helps with cataracts, as the lens of the eye is rich in Silica, and it is important in correcting any eye ailments and keeping infection at bay. In all these cases Silica is helpful; suck two tablets at least four times through the day and include Silica-rich foods in the diet. When there is sensitivity to bright light, Silica is again the answer. It is interesting to know that Silica comes from the seabed and rock crystal or quartz, and is used in the manufacture of glass lenses together with Calc. Fluor. Both are needed in our bodies, especially as we age, to maintain healthy lenses and eyes.

The ears

Deafness can be temporary or chronic, but Silica can most definitely be of assistance and comfort here. Deafness that is accompanied by heat, pain and inflammatory conditions responds well to Ferrum Phos. alternated with Kali. Mur. Suck two tablets of each frequently or make a hot drink with six tablets each of Silica, Kali. Mur. and Ferrum Phos. dissolved in a cup of hot water. Make the 'tea' again an hour or two later and continue until the condition improves; however, it is important to see your doctor.

Deafness can sometimes have a nervous cause, in which case Mag. Phos., Kali. Sulph. and Silica will calm and ease the situation. Dissolve six tablets of each in a cup of hot water, but again, check with your doctor. Hard wax in the ear can also cause deafness as well as noises in the ears. Suck two tablets each of Silica and Calc. Fluor. every 15 minutes to help dissolve or loosen the wax. If the condition does not improve, consult your doctor, as the ears may need to be syringed.

For complete deafness the best remedies are Kali. Sulph., Kali. Phos. and Silica, as well as vitamin C and vitamin A. Suck two tablets of each separately at least three times a day and consult an ENT specialist.

Oral health

When there are gum boils, bleeding gums, sores at the corners of the mouth, fever blisters, chapped bleeding lips, ulcerated or spongy gums, or if there is a mouth abscess, Silica comes to the rescue. It can be made into a paste and applied directly to the area. Crush four tablets in a teaspoon of hot water, work it into a paste and apply daily.

Also make a hot Silica 'tea' by dissolving 10 tablets in half a cup of hot water. Take small sips, swish the liquid around the mouth, hold for as long as possible and swallow. Do this frequently. Silica will 'ripen' an abscess and help to encourage its discharge, while also clearing and cleansing the area. After tooth extraction, sip the warm drink and hold it very gently in the mouth to help the healing process in the socket and gums – do not swish the fluid vigorously.

A good gargle to use when there are ulcerated spongy gums, halitosis and an unpleasant taste in the mouth is six tablets each of Silica, Calc.

Sulph. and Nat. Sulph. dissolved in half a glass of warm water. Take frequent sips and hold the fluid in the mouth to soothe and heal swiftly. Do not neglect this comforting and effective little ritual! It has been a noted treatment for gum boils, pyorrhoea and mouth ulcers for decades, and it always remains effective.

The respiratory system

Silica can help improve chest conditions such as pneumonia, bronchitis, tonsillitis and even asthma, which all involve mucus production and accumulation. A hot Silica 'tea' will go a long way towards healing and clearing the mucus build-up. To make the drink, dissolve eight Silica tablets in a cup of hot water and sip slowly two or three times a day. Remember that Silica heals and cleanses. If there is a tendency towards these conditions, add four Ferrum Phos. and four Kali. Mur. tablets to speed up the process as these three work well together. If you cannot get rid of a productive cough after a bout of flu, this trio will soon clear the lungs.

Silica skin cream for haemorrhoids, boils and scars

1 cup good aqueous cream
1 cup chopped fresh pennywort leaves and stems (*Centella asiatica*)
20 Silica, 10 Ferrum Phos. and 10 Calc. Fluor. tablets, crushed to a powder
2 teaspoons vitamin E oil

Simmer the aqueous cream and fresh pennywort in a double boiler, pressing the leaves down continuously with a stainless steel spoon for 20 minutes. Strain, add the tissue salt tablets crushed to a powder, and stir the cream thoroughly. Add the vitamin E oil and mix well. Spoon into glass jars and keep the excess in the fridge, labelled clearly.

Wash the area with warm water after going to the toilet and apply the cream. Be lavish in using this remarkable cream, as all itchy areas with cracks and bleeding will be soothed and healed quickly. During the winter months I add half a cup of calendula petals as this is a strong healing winter herb and is very well worth growing. Use the flowers when they are fully open.

The digestive system

A protruding stomach on a thin, elderly person often indicates lack of Silica, usually because the food is not being digested well. During our youth we can eat almost anything, but as the years add up, many people experience a burning sensation and discomfort during digestion, and poor absorption. Heartburn with discomfort and chronic diarrhoea can also be due to a lack of Silica. The latter often causes an irritated burning anus and haemorrhoids, and bleeding anal fissures. Constipation can also occur. However, the soothing Silica cream can be made easily to heal the area (see p.124).

The urinary system

When there is weakness with incontinence and painful urination, take two tablets each of Silica and Ferrum Phos. at least six times a day. If involuntary leaking occurs when coughing or sneezing, suck two tablets each of Ferrum Phos., Nat. Phos., Nat. Sulph. and Silica at least six times through the day.

Female problems

Silica will clear thick vaginal discharge, abscess formation and lumps in the vaginal wall, as well as boils, and it serves as a treatment for chronic cystitis. In all cases a hot Silica drink is soothing and helps to ease the discomfort of the infection. Dissolve 10 Silica tablets in a glass of hot water and sip slowly. Two or three glasses daily will clear chronic infections. In the case of hot flushes during menopause, take two Silica tablets 6–10 times through the day and night to calm and control the heat, and combine this with a Silica spritz-spray (10 tablets dissolved in a litre of cold water), which can be sprayed over the face, neck and arms.

Male problems

When there is chronic herpes infection, suck two tablets each of Ferrum Phos., Kali. Mur. and Silica six times a day. This helps to clear stubborn infection and slow-healing sores in the groin and inner thighs. Also apply Silica cream frequently (see recipe on p.124).

What you feel

Silica will help with anger and mood swings, irritability, obstinate or uncooperative behaviour, ill humour, general obstructive behaviour and aversion to work. When there is a debilitating 'gone' feeling and exhaustion with a sinking sensation, Silica comes to the rescue. Suck two tablets frequently until the shakiness goes.

12 Silica

Silica is a rescuer after shock, upsets or surgery, or during a long, cold winter. It is also an important energy salt – an energy manager – recommended when there is exhaustion, fatigue and listlessness. Managing energy is important as the ageing process presses upon us.

Silica also supports confidence, which is much needed as we age. Forgetfulness, reduced ability to work efficiently, a feeling of being incapable of performing a complicated task, lack of energy to start things, and general fear of mathematics, quick thinking and public speaking all call for Silica support.

When Silica is lacking we may become obsessed with details that almost drown us. Together with shortness of breath, this creates a vicious little circle of increasing worry and anxiety. However, Silica can ease, lift and steady us. The inclusion of a Silica drink or even a combination of all 12 tissue salts in one tablet (Combin 12) can begin to re-set our whole constitution.

Other ailments

When dust, talc, glaze powder or cement dust has been inhaled and lodged in the lungs and no amount of coughing can clear it, Silica is really necessary. Paint fumes, spray paints and potter's glazes can also damage the lungs. Suck two Silica tablets frequently until the breathing eases and consult a doctor if the discomfort persists.

If there are night sweats and copious perspiration, suck two Silica tablets every 20 minutes until the sweating eases and there is relief. You can also dissolve 10 crushed Silica tablets in a litre of cold water in a spritz-spray bottle and spray the body all over to lower the temperature.

A deficiency of Silica between the cerebrum and the cerebellum produces a mental condition in which thinking is difficult. Doctors Carey and Perry, who studied and wrote extensively on tissue salts, state that mental abstraction, despondence (often with depression) and general dislike and disgust with life, arise from insufficient Silica. According to them, quarrelling, warfare among nations and attraction to a fight of any kind is entirely due to disharmony of the brain cells. So Silica is the peacemaker – the reasonable, calming and quietening influence that helps to restore harmony and peace.

Silica is vitally important when there is alcoholism, and even in social drinking to control the need for more. Heavy alcohol consumption can lead to malnutrition, leaving the stomach lining raw and bleeding. This condition can be exacerbated by ingestion of painkillers. Take Silica with Mag. Phos. to ease this; two tablets of each sucked frequently will help you relax and sleep. It will also soothe restless legs and jerking limbs. After vaccinations or injections of any kind, Silica is the answer.

Secondary and complementary tissue salts

Calc. Sulph. and Mag. Phos. both work exceptionally well with Silica, which distributes calcium and magnesium. When there are rapid changes in the elderly person, these three need to be taken together daily – two tablets of each every morning and evening. Together they are great stabilisers of the whole body.

Herbs that contain Silica

Californian poppy (*Eschscholzia californica*): A winter annual, Californian poppy is a superb painkiller and a herb we should all be growing through the winter. It is a gentle antispasmodic and is particularly beneficial for mood swings, insomnia and anxiety. Make a tea from the petals and leaves as a night cap at the end of a tough day: pour a cup of boiling water over ¼ cup of the herb, let it draw for five minutes and stir well. The plant self-seeds abundantly and every autumn appears in many places in the garden, its fine, grey fern-like leaves marking the spot where a brilliance of silken orange flowers will appear in midwinter. It is an investment in the garden!

Comfrey (*Symphytum officinale*): I still think comfrey is a herbal miracle as it strengthens, builds and repairs bones like no other herb. However, it needs to be taken with caution, for only a short period, and in consultation with your doctor. Comfrey is rich in many minerals, particularly in Silica, and it is superb for knitting bones (hence it is often called 'knit-bone'). *Warning:* Take comfrey internally only under medical supervision, as the pyrrolizidine alkaloids in it have been linked to liver damage in rats. To make comfrey tea, pour a cup of boiling water over ¼ cup chopped fresh leaves, let the tea stand for five minutes, stir well, strain and sip. With your doctor's consent, take one cup a day no more than three times a week for four weeks to repair a fracture, for severe osteoporosis, or for pneumonia, flu and old wounds. Reduce sugar in the diet and include all the Silica herbs and foods listed here. Comfrey is rich in Silica and as an anti-ageing herb, it is beneficial when used correctly.

Dandelion (*Taraxacum officinale*): This herb is rich in Silica and its role in building the bones, teeth and nails is vital. Simply eating three fresh leaves with a salad daily is a valuable tonic for everyone aged over 50! It has a diuretic and antirheumatic action, and it serves as a liver and digestive tonic. Dandelion is one of the most necessary and vital anti-ageing herbs.

Horsetail (*Equisetum* species): This anti-inflammatory herb spreads easily in the garden, so be careful where you plant it as it even goes under stone pathways! Rich in Silica, it is best to take horsetail in homeopathic form.

Stinging nettle (*Urtica dioica*): This is an excellent diuretic and tonic herb, rich in vitamins A, B and C. Tea made from stinging nettle will clear uric acid from the joints, thus easing arthritis, rheumatism and gout. To make it, pour a cup of boiling water over ¼ cup fresh sprigs (use gloves to cut it); let the tea stand for five minutes, stir thoroughly, then strain and sip slowly. Have a cup daily.

Foods rich in Silica

In my long years of research into tissue salts I came across these words which I have never forgotten: 'Silica is present in all the tall grains, giving each stem the strength to bear the valuable mineral-rich seeds that form so great a part of humankind's food chain'. The grains include wheat, barley, maize, oats, rice, buckwheat, rye, spelt, sorghum, millet and sweet reed (a sorghum). All are Silica-rich and stand tall and unbreakable, even in strong winds, and can be grown easily as attractive plants in the garden. They can also be grown as mineral-rich sprouts on your kitchen windowsill!

Silica is also found abundantly in lentils, soya beans, spinach (especially spinach stems), lettuce, carrots, celery, chicory, apricots, lemons, oranges, guavas, pomegranates, apples and quinces.

When there are arthritic conditions, aching stiffness and rheumatism, avoid wheat bread and replace it with rye; also explore the delicious gluten-free potato-flour, rice-flour and almond-flour alternatives available.

Food sensitivities

As we age, we may find that sensitivities arise that we never had before, such as lactose intolerance, gluten intolerance, sensitivity to acid-forming foods, and so on. Keep a food diary to record, identify and eliminate foods that cause discomfort. Start your shopping trips in the fruit and vegetable area of your supermarket. It is here that you will build a healthy anti-ageing diet.

Silica fruit salad

Guavas
Pawpaw
Apricots
Berries in season
Banana
Grated apple
Figs
Pomegranates
Pineapple
Juice of 1 orange

Peel and chop the fruit and place it in a glass bowl; pour the fresh orange juice over it. Vary the fruit according to season. You can also add sunflower seeds, non-instant oats, chopped almonds and a little plain Bulgarian yoghurt, if desired.

Green mealie bread

Grow your own non-genetically modified mealies, and save the silk from those mealies for making into a tea to ease prostate problems.

6–8 mealies
3 tablespoons flour
2 level teaspoons baking powder
2 tablespoons soft butter
1 teaspoon Himalayan salt

Boil the mealies and cut the kernels off the cob to make four cups. Chop the kernels coarsely in a food processor. Add the remaining ingredients and mix well. Spoon the mixture into a buttered steaming bowl. Fold and tie a double layer of greaseproof paper over the top of the bowl and place it in a pot of water reaching $^2/_3$ of the way up the bowl. Bring the water to the boil and then simmer for two hours with the lid on. Once cool, remove the paper and run a knife around the bowl to loosen the bread. Serve with butter and fresh fruit – figs or apricots are my favourites!

Silica soup

SERVES 6

This hearty, easy-to-make soup is a delicious standby for those evenings when we do not feel like a heavy meal. Serve it warm with a little rye bread. It keeps well in a sealed container in the fridge.

2 cups sliced and chopped onions or leeks
Olive oil
1½ cups brown lentils
2 cups buckwheat sprouts
4 cups chopped spinach, stalks included
2 cups finely grated carrots
2 cups chopped celery
2 cups shredded lettuce
4 mealies, kernels cut off the cob
Juice of 2 lemons
1 teaspoon finely grated lemon zest
2 litres stock or water
Himalayan salt and red or black pepper

Brown the onions in the oil, then add all the other ingredients and stir well. I add three teaspoons of fresh thyme stripped off the stems for extra flavour, and two teaspoons of crushed coriander seeds. Simmer until all the ingredients are tender (at least one hour), and taste, as more lemon juice or salt may be needed. Serve piping hot and add a teaspoon or two of home-made chutney into each bowl for a full, rich flavour. I never tire of this power-packed soup. Once you've tried it, it's sure to become a standby for your family.

Perfectly lovely pomegranate

We grew up with pomegranate trees, and my grandmother used pomegranate juice to make cool-drink, ice cream lollies, and even pomegranate syrup with honey to have with rice pudding. Rice is rich in Silica; use only brown rice and make it with milk and honey and pour the wonderful pomegranate juice over it. It will be unforgettable!

To make my grandmother's pomegranate drink, carefully peel six fresh pomegranates and squash the juicy pips, using a spoon over a new sieve to release their juices. The fresh juice is beautifully sweet, but to be sure it was sweet enough, my grandmother always added a small spoon or two of honey and stirred it in well. Cover the jug with plastic wrap and store in the fridge until it is ready to serve, then serve with blocks of ice. It is more delicious than a bought cool-drink!

Do not throw the pomegranate seeds away. Save them and spread out onto a stainless steel tray to dry. Dried pomegranate seeds make a delicious spice with coriander and cumin. Keep the dried inner seeds in a screw-top glass bottle.

For festive occasions we made ice blocks with juicy pomegranate pips set into each little square of ice with a mint leaf and a blue borage flower. Try mixtures of garden fruit like strawberries or blackberries with pomegranate, or slices of ginger! Experiment to get maximum benefit from the freshest fruits.

Ailment chart

Note: Numbers in **semibold** next to an ailment refer to the number of the particular tissue salt(s) – see the box below. A plus (+) sign denotes combinations of tissue salts. Refer to the main text (page in brackets) for the suggested dosage or method of application and other important information.

The 12 Tissue Salts

1. **Calc. Fluor.** – *Calcarea Fluorata* (p.13)

2. **Calc. Phos.** – *Calcarea Phosphoricum* (p.24)

3. **Calc. Sulph.** – *Calcarea Sulphurica* (p.34)

4. **Ferrum Phos.** – *Ferrum Phosphoricum* (p.43)

5. **Kali. Mur.** – *Kalium Muriaticum* (p.52)

6. **Kali. Phos.** – *Kalium Phosphoricum* (p.62)

7. **Kali. Sulph.** – *Kalium Sulphuricum* (p.71)

8. **Mag. Phos.** – *Magnesia Phosphorica* (p.80)

9. **Nat. Mur.** – *Natrum Muriaticum* (p.89)

10. **Nat. Phos.** – *Natrum Phosphoricum* (p.101)

11. **Nat. Sulph.** – *Natrum Sulphuricum* (p.113)

12. **Silica** – *Silicea* (p.120)

A

Aches and pains **12** (p.120)

Acne **2** (p.29); **3** (p.35); **5** (p.57); **9** (p.90); **10** (p.108)

Adenoids, swollen **5** (p.54)

Age spots **3** (p.38)

Aggressiveness **2+5+8** (p.30)

Agitation **8** (p.84)

Alcohol, heavy consumption, raw and bleeding stomach lining **8+12** (p.126)

over indulgence **9** (p.95)

Alcoholism 12 (p.126)
Alopecia 9 (p.95)
Anaemia 4+9 (p.48)
Anal fissures and cracks 2 (p.28);
9 (p.93); 1+4+12 (p.124 and 125)
Anal, itching 10 and 4+10
(p.102)
Aneurism, threatened 1+4 (p.48)
Anger 10 (p.107); 12 (p.125)
Angina pectoris 6+8 (p.64)
Ankles, itchy 10 and 4+10 (p.102)
sprained, twisted 1 (p.14)
swollen 9 (p.95)
Ankylosing spondylitis 12 (p.121)
Anxiety 7 (p.75); 4+7+8+9+12
(p.94)
reduction of 2+8 (p.85)
Appetite, restore 3 (p.38)
Arthritis 8 (p.85); 4+10 and
10+11+12 (p.102)
chronic 12 (p.121)
pain 9 (p.95)
Asthma 1+4+5+9+11 (p.55); 7
(p.73); 9 (p.95); 11 (p.115); 12,
4+5+12 (p.124)
chronic, nervous, wheezing,
distress 6+8 (p.65)
Astigmatism 4+6+8 (p.63)
Athlete's foot 7+11 (p.117)

B

Back discomfort and pain due to
bladder weakness 1+7 (p.18)
pain lower, 1 (p.14); 8 (p.85)
slipped discs 1 (p.14)
Backache 4+12 (p.48); 4+5+8+10
(p.52)
Balance, lack of 8 (p.85)
Behaviour, erratic 1 (p.19)

Belching 1 (p.17); 2 (p.28) 2+8+10
(p.28); 2+4 (p.45); 5 (p.55); 7 (p.74);
9 (p.92)
sour gas 10 (p.105)
Bell's palsy 6 (p.63)
Bladder, complaints 3 (p.38)
strengthen 1 (p.18)
Blisters 4+5 (p.57); 9 (p.89)
Bloating 5 (p.55); 7 (p.74); 9 (p.92)
Blood poisoning 7 (p.75)
Blood pressure, high 4+6 (p.64)
low 4+10+11 (p.117)
Blood, keep alkaline 8 (p.83)
Body odour 6+10+12 (p.65)
Body, stabiliser 3+8+12 (p.127)
Boils 3 (p.34)
infected 3 (p.34)
slow healing on legs, groin and
hip joint 3 (p.37)
Bones, aches and pains, poor
circulation 2 (p.25)
chilliness, aching, numbness
2+4 (p.25)
discomfort in 7+8 (p.75)
fragile 12 (p.121)
pain 1 (p.14)
'spurs' 1 (p.13)
strengthen 1 (p.13)
ulcers, abscesses with
restlessness 2 (p.25)
weak 12 (p.120)
Bowel, distended pockets 1 (p.17)
Brain fatigue 6 (p.63)
Breasts, cysts 1 (p.18)
Breath, bad 6+10+12 (p.65); 11
(p.116); 3+11+12 (p.123)
gasping 6+8 (p.65)
shortness 4+5 (p.47), 4 (p.48)
sweeten 1 (p.16)

133

hot, itchy 4+10 (p.105); 9 (p.95)
infections 5 (p.54)
loosen wax 1+12 (p.123)
middle, infection 1+12 (p.16)
middle, inflammation of, 8 (p.81)
polyps 7 (p.72)
redness and soreness of outer 4 (p.44)
ringing 8 (p.81)
tinnitus 6 (p.64)
Eczema, burning, dry, sensitive 3 (p.34)
  infected 6+8 (p.65)
  lotion 9+10+11 (p.114)
  weeping 4 (p.57); 7 (p.72); 9 (p.89)
Elbow, inflammation in joint 5 (p.58)
  stiffness in the joint, pain 1 (p.14)
Eliminating 3 (p.34)
Endocrine, imbalance 9 (p.95)
Energy spark 10+11+12 (p.117)
  lack of 2 (p.24); 6 (p.66); 9 (p.95)
Epilepsy 1+4 (p.48)
Exhaustion 8 (p.84); 8 (p.85); 12 (p.126)
  nervous 2+4+6 (p.66)
  with debilitating sinking sensation 12 (p.125)
Eyes, blurred, weakened or distorted vision 6 (p.63)
  blurred vision, focus delay, nervous tics, ache, itchiness, irritation, tears 1 (p.15)
  discharge 5 (p.54)
  dull, blurred sight, drooping eyelids 6+8 (p.81)
  fatigue 6, 6+8, 4+6+8 (p.63)

infection 3 (p.35)
itchy, sore, red scratchy 4+8 (p.81)
itchy, watery, bags, puffiness, scratchy, dry, weak 9 (p.91)
oversensitive to light, twitches, red irritated, aching stiffness behind eyeball 2 (p.25)
pain 6+8 (p.63)
sore, red, watery, painful, dry, sandpapery 4 (p.44)
spontaneous tic 8 (p.81)
sunken, deep, red eyelids, styes, itching, sensitivity to bright light 12 (p.122)
watery 4+5 (p.54)

F

Face pulling 6+8 (p.81)
Face, blotchy red, no fever 10 (p.107)
Faintness 4 (p.43)
Fatigue 3 (p.39); 2+4+6 (p.47); 8 (p.84); 12 (p.120); 12 (p.126)
  chronic 2+4+6 (p.66); 12 (p.121)
Fear 2+5+8 (p.30); 11, 6+11 (p.116)
  ageing related 2+4+6+12 (p.66)
  of performing tasks 12 (p.126)
Feet, burning 3 (p.37)
  smelly 6+10+12 (p.65)
  swelling with pain 12 (p.120)
Fever 4 (p.48)
  high 7 (p.76)
  with blocked nose 4+4+6+11 (p.44)
Fever blisters 4 (p.44); 9 (p.91); 12 (p.123)
Fibroids 1 (p.18)
Fingers and toes, itchy 10 and 4+10 (p.102)

after eating 10 (p.107)
result of intense stress and
anxiety 5 (p.56)
Heartbeat, irregular 8 (p.84); 9
(p.95)
Heartburn 2+4 (p.45); 8 (p.82); 9
(p.92); 12 (p.125)
repeated 10 (p.105)
Heels cracked, calloused 1 (p.18); 3
(p.37)
Helplessness 1 (p.19); 2+5+8 (p.30)
with heart palpitations 2+5+8
(p.30)
Hepatitis 5 (p.58)
Herpes, chronic infection, men
4+5+12 (p.125)
Hiatus hernia 1 (p.17)
Hiccups 1 (p.17); 8 (p.82)
Hip joint, inflammation 5 (p.58)
Hips, sore 1 (p.14)
Hives 9 (p.89)
Hoarseness 2+9 and 2+4 (p.30)
Hodgkin's disease 1 (p.18)
Hopelessness 1 (p.19); 6+11
(p.117)
Hot flushes 7 (p.74); 12 (p.125)
Hunger, constant 10 (p.105)
pangs 8 (p.82)
Hypoglycaemia 10 (p.108)

I

Immune booster 2 (p.30)
Immune system, stimulate 4+5
(p.47); 6 (p.68)
Impatience 11 (p.117)
Incontinence 4+6 and 4+10 (p.46)
Indigestion 8 (p.82); 9 (p.92)
burning 2+8+10 (p.28); 3 (p.38); 6
(p.64); 11 (p.115)

Infections, old, lingering 4+5+7 (p.58)
Insect bites 9 (p.89)
Insomnia 2+4+6+8+10 (p.48); 6
(p.66); 9 (p.95)
Instability 1 (p.19)
Irritability 1 (p.19); 2+4+6 (p.47);
7 (p.75); 10 (p.107); 11 (p.117); 12
(p.125)
Irritable bowel syndrome 1 (p.17);
2+6+11 (p.28); 8 (p.82)

J

Jaundice 5 (p.58); 10 (p.106)
Joints, aching 2+4+12 (p.25); 3
(p.38); 7+8 (p.75); 10 and 10+11+12
(p.102)
fungoid inflammation 7 (p.75)
hot sore swollen 4+9+10 (p.50)
pain, stiffness 4+5+8+10 (p.52)
stiff 11 (p.114)
strengthen 1 (p.13)
that crack audibly 9 (p.95)

K

Kidney stones developing 4+6+8
(p.83)
passing 4+6+8+11 (p.83)
Kidney, aches, complaints 3 (p.38)
inflammation 4+6+9 (p.47)
pain 4+12 (p.48)
Knee, weight-bearing problem,
slips out of socket easily, aches 1
(p.14)

L

Lassitude 11 (p.117)
Legs, swollen 9 (p.95)
swollen, aching 12 (p.120)
ulcers 3 (p.37)

weakness **10** and **10+11+12**
(p.102)
Leucorrhoea **4+5** (p.56); **7** (p.74)
Libido, decreased **4+7+8+9+12** (p.94)
Ligaments, slip easily **1** (p.14)
Limb, jerking during sleep **9** (p.95);
12 (p.127)
    lower, burning **3** (p.37)
Lips, bleeding **12** (p.123)
    cracked **1** (p.15)
    dry, cracked **1+9** (p.91)
    twitches and spasms **6+8**
    (p.81)
Listlessness **3** (p.39); **12** (p.126)
Liver, cleanser after medication **3+8**
(p.38)
    congestion **5** (p.55)
    discomfort **10+11** (p.106)
Liverish condition, over-acidic
10+11 (p.117)
Lockjaw **8** (p.81)
Lower back, ease discomfort **1** (p.13)
Lumbago **12** (p.120)
Lupus **5** (p.57)
Lymph glands, knotty, nodules,
swollen **1** (p.18)
    swollen neck **5** (p.54)

M

Malaria, support **11**, **4+6+11**, **4+11**
(p.116)
Measles **7** (p.72)
Melancholy **11**, **6+11** (p.116)
Memory loss **2+5+8** (p.30)
    poor **6** (p.63)
Menopausal (post) discomfort and
bloating **4+5+9+10** (p.56)
Menopause, hot flushes **7** (p.74); **12**
(p.125)

hot flushes, vertigo, fluid
retention, anxiety **4+6** (p.47)
    problems **2** (p.30)
Menstruation, cramps **4+8** (p.47)
    excessive bleeding **4+5** (p.47)
    irregular, excessive bleeding **4**
    (p.47)
    painful **4+5+9+10** (p.56)
    painful, large clots **4+6+8** (p.83)
Mental deterioration **6** (p.66)
Metabolism, regulate **9+10+11** (p.117)
Migraine, sinus-related **7** (p.73)
Mood swings **8** (p.84); **12** (p.125)
Mood, calming **1** (p.19); **12** (p.126)
    heavy **2+4+6** (p.66)
    lift spirits **2+6** (p.29); **6+8** (pp.84
    and 85); **9** (p.94); **2+6+11** (p.117)
Moodiness **2+5+8** (p.30)
Mosquito bites **8** (p.85); **9** (p.89)
    infected **3** (p.35)
Mouth, bitter taste **11** (p.116)
    dry **1** (p.15)
    infections **3+4** (p.36)
    minor problems **2** (p.27)
    sores at corner of **1** (p.15)
    sores at corners, abscess **12**
    (p.123)
    ulcers **3** (p.36); **4** (p.44); **1+9**
    (p.91); **3+11+12** (p.124)
    ulcers, white **5** (p.58)
    unpleasant taste **3+11+12** (p.123)
Mucous membranes, congested **4+5**
(p.47)
Mucus, build-up **7** (p.72)
    clearing build-up **12** and **4+5+12**
    (p.124)
    clearing out **3** (p.34); **3+4+7**
    (p.75)
Multiple sclerosis **6** (p.66)

Rectum, burning sensation 7 (p.74)
Reflux, sour 10 (p.105)
Respiratory problems 5 (p.58)
Retinitis 4 (p.44)
Rheumatic lameness 1+4 (p.48)
Rheumatism 2 (p.25); 4+12 (p.48);
  8 (p.85)
  chronic 12 (p.121)
  painful 7 (p.75)
Rhinitis 9 (p.95)

S

Sadness 1 (p.19); 7 (p.75);
  4+7+8+9+12 (p.94)
Scabs, crusty 11 (p.114)
Scalp, blisters and crusts 5 (p.58)
  itchy 4+6+8 (p.65); 10 (p.102)
Scarlet fever 7 (p.72)
Scars 12 (p.121)
Sciatic, nerve pain 8 (p.85)
  pain, down back of leg 11
  (p.115)
Sciatica 12 (p.120)
Sensitivity, noise 6 (p.63); 7 (p.75)
Shingles 5 (p.57); 6+8 (p.65); 5+6+9
  with 2+4 (p.90)
Shins, itchy 10 and 4+10 (p.102)
Shock, after 12 (p.126)
Sighing, frequent 2+6 (p.29)
Sinusitis 4+5 (p.54); 9 (p.95)
Skeletal pain and discomfort 12
  (p.121)
Skin, chafed 4+5 (p.57)
  cysts, bumps 1 (p.18)
  discharge 7 (p.76)
  dry 3 (p.37)
  dry facial 9 (p.90)
  eruptions 3 (p.35)
  irritated 9+10+11 (p.114)

itching 5 (p.58); 8 (p.85); 11
  (p.114)
oily and acne 9 (p.90)
pale, pasty, spots, adult acne
  2 (p.29)
rash, heat bumps 4+10 (p.102)
spots, rashes, red, itchy 7 (p.72)
suppurating sores 3 (p.35)
thin, fragile 12 (p.121)
tone and restore elasticity 2+6
  (p.67)
unhealthy, infected spots, oily
  patches 3 (p.34)
Sleep, lack of 2+6 (p.29)
  poor 8 (p.84)
  restless 10 (p.105)
  waking with anxiety or despair
  2+3+6 (p.39)
  worries, grief, anxiety, disturbing
  dreams 1+6+12 (p.19)
Sluggishness 2 (p.30)
Smell, loss of 8 (p.82)
  sense of compromised 7+9 (p.92)
Sneezing, repetitive 9 (p.95)
Sores, festering 5 (p.57)
Spasm, relief from 2+8 (p.80)
Spine, curvature 2+12 (p.25)
Sprains 4 (p.48)
St Vitis dance 8 (p.80)
Stammering, spasmodic 6+8 (p.81)
Stiffness 4+12 (p.48)
  chronic 9 (p.95)
Stomach, burning sensation 5 (p.55)
  churning 10 (p.105)
  pain after eating 2 (p.28)
  ulcer 3 (p.38); 10 (p.105)
Stool, unsuccessful desire to pass 2
  (p.28)
Stress 8 (p.85)

Stroke, after 4+6+8 (p.66); 12 (p.122)
Suffocation, feeling of due to
  enlargement of goitre 2 (p.30)
Sunburn 4+5 (p.57); 8 (p.85); 9 (p.89)
Sunstroke 9 (p.93)
Surgery, after 12 (p.126)
Swallowing, difficulty 7 (p.75)
Sweating, from head at night 2 (p.30)
  heavy 9 (p.95)
  palms 2 (p.30)
Swelling 8 (p.85)
Synovitis 12 (p.121)
Syphilis 9 (p.95)

T

Taste, sense of compromised 7+9
  (p.92)
Tearfulness 9 (p.95)
Teeth, decay 2 (p.26)
  feeling loose 1 (p.15)
  grinding 10 (p.105)
  sensitivity 1 (p.16)
  sensitivity to cold or touch 8 (p.82)
  strengthening 2 (p.26)
Temper, quick 7 (p.75)
  short 1 (p.19); 11 (p.117)
  tantrums 6 (p.63)
Temples, throbbing 12 (p.122)
Tendons, no elasticity, hardened,
  tumours on 1 (p.14)
  slip easily 1 (p.14)
Testicles, swelling 4+5 (p.56)
Thinking, difficult 12 (p.126)
  incoherent 2+5+8 (p.30)
Throat, clear frog in, burning 2+4+9
  (p.30)
Throat, constricted feeling 8 (p.82)
  discharge 7 (p.76)
  phlegmy 5 (p.54)

sore 3+7 (p.37)
sore, ulcers 4 (p.44)
  spasm 6+8 (p.82)
Throat-clearing, while speaking
  2+9 and 2+4 (p.30)
Thrush, mouth 5 (p.54)
Thyroid 7 (p.76)
Tinnitus 4+6+8 (p.64)
Tobacco craving 2 (p.24) 2 (p.30)
Toes and fingers, itchy 10 and 4+10
  (p.102)
Tongue, marks on 1+9 (p.91)
  red inflamed 4 (p.44)
  yellowish coating 10
  (p.105)
Tonsillitis 3+7 (p.37); 12, 4+5+12
  (p.124)
Tonsils, inflamed 3+4+5 (p.45)
  swollen 5 (p.54)
Tooth, extraction 12 (p.123)
Toothache 4+8 (p.44)
Touchiness 8 (p.84)
Travel formula for stomach
  1+3+5+7+12 (p.38)
Typhoid 7 (p.75)
Typhus 7 (p.75)

U

Underarm, itching and sweating 10
  (p.107)
Unsteadiness 12 (p.122)
Urethra, strengthen 1 (p.18)
  stricture 8 (p.83)
Urination, burning after 4+6 and
  4+10 (p.46)
  constant urge 4+6+9 (p.47)
  difficulty 8 (p.83)
  frequent 9 (p.93); 10 and 4+10
  (p.107)

involuntary leaking when
coughing 4+10+11+12 (p.125)
on coughing or sneezing 10 and
formula 2+6+9+10 (p.106)
painful retention 6+8 (p.83)
painful with incontinence 4+12
(p.125)
strain 6+8 (p.83)
Uterine cramps 4+7+8+9+12 (p.94)

V

Vaginal, discharge, abscess, lumps,
boils 12 (p.125)
discharge 7 (p.76)
itching and discharge 10, wash
4+10 (p.105); 11 (p.116)
Vaginitis 4+5 (p.56)
Varicose veins 1 (p.17); 4 (p.48); 7
(p.74); 9 (p.93)
slow-healing and painful 3
(p.37)
Varicosities, throbbing with cold
feet, ulcerated 3 (p.36)
Vertigo 2+4+8+9 (p.30); 4 (p.43); 9
(p.93); 12 (p.122)

Vision, blurred 8 (p.81)
focus delay, nervous tic 1 (p.15)
Vitiligo 7 (p.72)
Voice, croaky and uneven 3+4+5
(p.45)
Vomiting 1 (p.17); 2 (p.28); 4+6
(p.45)
green bile 11 (p.116)
occasional of sour foods 10 (p.105)
with griping pains 8 (p.82)

W

Warts 9 (p.95); 12 (p.121)
Weariness 1 (p.13); 5 (p.58); 12
(p.120)
Weeping 2+6 (p.29)
Weight loss, due to grief or stress
2 (p.30)
Wheezing, thick phlegm 11 (p.115)
Willpower, lack of 2 (p.24)
Worry 2+4+6 (p.63)
ageing related 2+4+6+12 (p.66)
imagined problems 3 (p.39)
Wrists, bony outgrowths, cysts,
injuries on 1 (p.14)

In the end, it's not the years in your life that count. It's the life in your years.

Abraham Lincoln